Understanding Health Psychology Through the Works of Stephen King

Not just your regular textbook, this unique book uses popular culture as a teaching tool by taking the work of Stephen King, America's top horror writer, to illustrate concepts that are essential to health psychology. This book uses his storytelling and character development to illustrate the science of how psychology "gets under the skin" to impact physical health. It examines the history of health psychology and the biopsychosocial perspective, the biology of stress and emotion, the science of behavior change, structural (social) influences on health, personality and sleep science, the role of psychology in disease, and the evidence of the mind-body connection.

This book provides definitions of many health psychology concepts and uses the works of Stephen King to couch them in an easy-to-understand context. The intrinsic enjoyment of relating to a popular fiction writer is used to present the most recent research in the field, including work in the neuroscience of health psychology and the science of intervention. From explorations of the placebo and nocebo effects in *Holly* and *Thinner*, to the socioecological impacts on health in *The Running Man* and the power of adverse childhood experiences in *The Body*, this book provides a wide-reaching overview of health psychology that can provide context for psychology students as well as student engagement opportunities.

Accompanied by supplementary teaching materials, this engaging read is designed to motivate undergraduate health psychology students and educators. It is also intended for King's Constant Readers – those who can't get enough of the world of Stephen King.

Crista Crittenden, PhD, MPH, LSW, is currently special faculty in psychology with a joint position at both Carnegie Mellon University in Pittsburgh and Carnegie Mellon University in Qatar. She teaches a wide range of courses, from introductory cognitive psychology lectures to upper-level clinical and health psychology seminars. She is also a licensed social worker who provides supervised pro bono therapy, focusing on cognitive behavioral therapy and psychodynamic psychotherapy. She earned her bachelor's degree in brain and cognitive science from the University of Rochester, her master's degrees in public health and social work from the University of Rochester School of Medicine and Dentistry and from the University of Pittsburgh, respectively, and her PhD in psychology from Carnegie Mellon University.

Understanding Health Psychology Through the Works of Stephen King

Getting Under Your Skin

Crista Crittenden

Routledge
Taylor & Francis Group
NEW YORK AND LONDON

Designed cover image: Getty Images

First published 2026
by Routledge
605 Third Avenue, New York, NY 10158

and by Routledge
4 Park Square, Milton Park, Abingdon, Oxon, OX14 4RN

Routledge is an imprint of the Taylor & Francis Group, an informa business

ISBN: 9781032802084 (hbk)
ISBN: 9781032802077 (pbk)
ISBN: 9781003495994 (ebk)

DOI: 10.4324/9781003495994

Typeset in Times New Roman
by codeMantra

Access the Support Material: www.routledge.com/9781032802077

Thank you to Sheldon Cohen for the facts and Stephen King for the fiction.

Contents

Preface

Thank you so much for picking up this book – I hope that you found the title intriguing and are here to get some learning! As far as I can see, this book has three main audiences: those who want to learn about health psychology, those who want to teach health psychology, and Constant Readers.

Those Who Want to Learn about Health Psychology

At some point, I was an undergraduate student taking an intro to health psychology course, learning about these concepts for the first time. Then I was a graduate student learning to become an expert in these topics. This book was written with all levels of learning in mind. It provides the foundational material for understanding health psychology as well as some more specific and thought-provoking material for those going beyond the basics. No matter what level you are approaching it with, I hope that you find Stephen King's framework fun and engaging and that it keeps you on your toes! The point is to learn the material and apply it in ways that might not be apparent in a simple Health Psych 101 course.

Those Who Want to Teach Health Psychology

No matter what subject you teach, teaching is getting harder with each passing semester. The hot topic on campuses throughout the world these past few years has, of course, been artificial intelligence (AI). How ChatGPT and the like make our roles as instructors, who are trying to encourage independent thought and critical analysis, more difficult (or easier, as some may argue) has been on everyone's mind. One of the main motivations for this out-of-the-box textbook is that we can approach health psychology in a way that may not be easily replicated by large language models (LLMs), so that students can truly put their own thinking and understanding to the test. At the end of each chapter, instructors will find assignment questions that involve critical thinking about Stephen King's books, movies, and TV shows and applying them to health psychology. It is hoped that this approach will make students more intrinsically (and entertainingly) motivated to do their own work and research and thus take more from health psychology than a general textbook would allow. And I hope it is fun for the instructors as well!

Constant Readers

If you are a Constant Reader, then you know what I am referring to, and nothing more needs to be said. For those of you who don't know, "Constant Readers" is how Stephen King refers to those whom he believes are consistently reading his books. He has an amazingly large and wide-reaching fanbase. It covers those who love movies like *The Shawshank Redemption* and *Stand By Me* to those who may devour Marvel Comics' *The Stand*, to those who read each and every King's book on the day it is released. Some Constant Readers, like me, may be late to the party, but are ready to soak up all things King to make up for the time they have missed. This book is for all Constant Readers or soon-to-be Constant Readers. I hope it brings a new level to your enjoyment of King's work, so that you may rediscover some of your old favorites and appreciate the new works to come.

A Note about Spoilers

Whenever I am addressing a certain work by Stephen King, I provide a very limited summary – so that those who have never read the book, or those who haven't read it in a while, understand or remember the basic premise and characters. As best I could, I tried to leave out spoilers – I would hate to be the person who ruined a key surprise or discovery for you! Unfortunately, some of my discussions about health psychology concepts revolve around key plot points, and you may experience a spoiler or two. So please proceed with caution!

Acknowledgments

I just want to give a quick shout out to my social support systems and the people who provide me with my healthy levels of social integrations (please read this book to find out more!). First, thanks to the advising queens of psychology – you know who you are. Thanks of course to my transglobal friend groups – the Swissvale Opera Club of Pittsburgh and the Hibachi Brunch Club of Doha – I love you all. I could never be where I am today without the unconditional love and support of my mom – you have given me everything I needed to live an amazing life. And while all of those mentioned above have put up with so much during the writing of this book, the person who put up with the most was my husband. Husband – I apologize for all you had to suffer through as I wrote and I wrote. You are the best – don't ever forget that my life is immeasurably better with you in it.

Acronyms and Abbreviations

ACC – Anterior Cingulate Cortex
ACE – Adverse Childhood Experience
ACTH – Adrenocorticotropic Hormone
ADHD – Attention-Deficit/Hyperactivity Disorder
ANS – Autonomic Nervous System
APC – Antigen-Presenting Cell
APS – American Psychosomatic Society
AUD – Alcohol Use Disorder
BMI – Body Mass Index
BP – Blood Pressure
CAR – Cortisol Awakening Response
CBT – Cognitive Behavioral Therapy
CBT-I – Cognitive Behavioral Therapy for Insomnia
CHD – Coronary Heart Disease
CNS – Central Nervous System
CR – Conditioned Response
CS – Conditioned Stimulus
CRH – Corticotropin-Releasing Hormone
CRP – C-Reactive Protein
CVD – Cardiovascular Disease
DSM – *Diagnostic and Statistical Manual of Mental Disorders*
DV – Dependent Variable
DZ – Dizygotic
ENS – Enteric Nervous System
ESWS – End-Systolic Wall Stress
ETS – Environmental Tobacco Smoke
GSR – Galvanic Skin Response
HBM – Health Belief Model
HPA – Hypothalamic-Pituitary-Adrenal
HR – Heart Rate
IQ – Intelligence Quotient
IV – Independent Variable

LEO – Law Enforcement Officer
MDD – Major Depressive Disorder
MZ – Monozygotic
NREM – Non-Rapid Eye Movement
NS – Neutral Stimulus
PCS3 – Pittsburgh Cold Study 3
PEFR – Peak Expiratory Flow Rate
PMBC – Pittsburgh Mind-Body Center
PNI – Psychoneuroimmunology
PNS – Peripheral Nervous System
PSS – Perceived Stress Scale
PTSD – Post-Traumatic Stress Disorder
RCT – Randomized Controlled Trial
REM – Rapid Eye Movement
SAM – Sympatho-Adrenal-Medullary
SBSM – Society for Biopsychosocial Science and Medicine
SCN – Suprachiasmatic Nucleus
SES – Socioeconomic Status
SI – Social Integration
SK – Stephen King
SNS – Sympathetic Nervous System
SUD – Substance Use Disorder
SWS – Slow Wave Sleep
TCM – Takotsubo Cardiomyopathy
TPB – Theory of Planned Behavior
TTM – Transtheoretical Model
UR – Unconditioned Response
US – Unconditioned Stimulus
VTA – Ventral Tegmental Area
WHO – World Health Organization

1 Getting Under Your Skin

A Shining Introduction

My Introduction to Stephen King

Many of you reading this might have once been like me, or maybe you still are – a pompous jerk. That is, you stuck your nose up at Stephen King. When I was in my teens and twenties, I refused to read Stephen King. It was all too "plebeian." Give me your Hemingways, your Garcia-Marquezs, your Atwoods. But PLEASE – Stephen King? Never. I wish I could go back and kick my own butt, but alas, time travel eludes us. How many hours of pleasurable reading did I miss? Let us not dwell – let us just appreciate that we are here now and that we recognize that Stephen King is so much more than just a popular horror writer. In fact, he may be the key to helping us learn about and understand the field of health psychology.

I first got over myself when I was in graduate school, getting my PhD in psychology at Carnegie Mellon University in Pittsburgh, Pennsylvania. It was my last year in a five-and-a-half-year sentence, and I was desperately trying to finish my dissertation. My dissertation was meant to be a culmination of everything I had learned about health psychology over half a decade of study. Things were not going well. Everything distracted me, everything was an excuse to not work on the one thing that would get me out of the purgatory of a PhD program. Recognizing that I needed a distraction-free environment, I rashly decided to book a few nights at the Holiday Inn in downtown Johnstown, PA, a little less than two hours away from Pittsburgh. Here, I could just devote the distraction-free time I needed to write.

For those of you who don't know, Johnstown is the location of one of the biggest man-made disasters in the United States – the Johnstown flood. In 1889, the South Fork Dam broke, flooding Johnstown and killing over 2,000 people.[1] I will spare you the details, but just say it is unclear whether the city ever got over the disaster, and it seems haunted by events of the past. Some of you may be starting to see where I am going with this.

While struggling with my dissertation alone in my hotel room, I decided it would be a good idea to take periodic breaks to read something completely unrelated to the work I was doing. Why did I pick this point in my life to finally pick up a Stephen King book? I have no idea. I have the sneaking suspicion it had something to do with the book being about a struggling writer holed up in a haunted hotel. Yes, I decided to start reading *The Shining* (see summary Box 1.1).

DOI: 10.4324/9781003495994-1

⚠ **[Spoiler Alert]**

Box 1.1 *The Shining*

After *Carrie* and *Salem's Lot* came King's third novel, *The Shining*. The "shining" itself refers to the psychic powers experienced by Danny Torrence, the five-year-old son of Jack Torrence, whom the book is focused on. When we meet Jack at the beginning of the book, he is having a hard go of it. He has recently been let go from his job as an English teacher at a pretty posh New England school, after his explosive temper had led him to assault a student. He is also trying to write a play, as well as hang on to his sobriety, and is struggling with both. In need of money and time to work on the play, he accepts the position of winter caretaker at the Overlook Hotel, high in the mountains of Colorado.

Despite the suggestions of the hotel manager to not bring his family, Jack decides to bring his wife, Wendy, and son, Danny, to spend the long, secluded winter months with him at the Overlook. For approximately six months, it will be just the three of them, living in the mostly snowed-in hotel, with the main goal being to keep the furnace going in rotating sections of the hotel so that the pipes don't freeze.

Sounds easy, right? The hotel chef, Dick Halloran, has made sure they have more than enough food to hold them over for the winter. He has also made sure that Danny, who has the same "shine" that Dick has, knows to watch out for the hotel and to use his psychic abilities should Danny find himself in trouble. Dick leaves the Torrences behind, off to a sweet winter gig in Florida. But of course, he has misgivings, as he has come to believe that the Overlook is haunted.

It is not just the hotel that is haunted – Jack Torrence is haunted as well. Haunted with the memories of his childhood, his early successes as a writer, his hard-drinking days, and the bursts of anger that have led him to move his entire family to a secluded hotel. As the winter closes in, Jack starts to feel the pressure – the pressure of completing his play, of caring for his family, of staying sober, and of dealing with the Overlook and its many needs and demands.

And the hotel does indeed start to get demanding. The hotel has a sordid history, with deaths abounding – from gangsters to heiresses to the previous caretaker and his family. It now seems that those departed do the work of the hotel, and the hotel wants Danny. Danny has powerful abilities to read minds, see the future, and understand others more than they understand themselves. Danny is strong, and so is his mom, so the hotel has chosen Jack to be its conduit to Danny. The hotel, sensing Jack's weaknesses, plies him with booze and accolades, and he becomes the hand by which the hotel works.

Unfortunately for Danny and Wendy, what the hotel wants Jack to do is kill them, specifically with a roque (croquet-like) mallet. Sensing the trouble,

Danny screams down the psychic pipeline to Dick in Florida, begging him to come and help. As Jack becomes progressively more violent, Danny and Wendy fight in any way they can, recognizing that the man chasing them through the hotel is no longer their husband and father, but some manifestation of the evil of the hotel.

Things get pretty desperate once Jack critically injures Wendy and sets his sights on Danny. After a perilous journey from Florida in which universal forces tried to stop Dick from getting to the hotel, he arrives at a gruesome scene of Wendy bleeding and broken, and Danny being pursued by his dad, who, in all actuality, should be dead given his injuries from his fight with Wendy. In a last moment of fight and clarity, Jack tells Danny to get out of the hotel. Danny also remembers that his dad has not done his most important caretaking duty – relieving the pressure of the basement boiler, and the hotel is probably going to blow. Danny finds his mom and Dick, and they get out just in time to watch the hotel – and Jack Torrence – go up in flames.

On the second night of my Holiday Inn stay, I was getting far into the book (and not so far into my dissertation). And I was getting scared. I mean more scared than I have ever been. I could feel my body experiencing the sympathetic nervous system activation we associate with "fight or flight." I could feel my blood pressure increasing, and my face felt red. My palms began to sweat. I could feel my heart racing – it was telling me to make sure I locked the hotel door – for the 20th time. The door was locked! I wasn't in any danger. But my body was reacting as if survival was not a foregone conclusion of my weekend at the Johnstown Holiday Inn.

How was Stephen King able to get under my skin and cause such a strong biological reaction? It was just a book – words on a piece of paper. Words that were written over 30 years ago, at that! Yet there I was, deep in it. It was then that I realized Stephen King was not just a horror writer – he was a person who could elicit emotions and influence my psychological state in such a way that I could biologically change. His work, and what he is able to do with his words, is the embodiment of the ideas of health psychology.

What Is Health Psychology?

Health psychology, as will be discussed in this book, is the scientific endeavor of connecting psychology to physical health. More specifically, it focuses on the biopsychosocial model of health and illness. The biopsychosocial model says we need to not just focus on the physical or biological components of our health but also look at the psychological and social factors that are at play. The biopsychosocial model is attributed to the work of George Engel at my undergraduate and graduate alma mater, the University of Rochester (Go Yellowjackets!). The idea of the biopsychosocial model is in sharp contrast to the biomedical model, which we will discuss more about in Chapter 2. What you need to know at this point is that the biomedical model says that health is of the body only, whereas the biopsychosocial model says that health is of the body and mind. And this is where Stephen King comes into the picture.

Box 1.2 What Is Health?

We keep speaking of health, but what does it actually mean? For the purposes of this book, we will use the World Health Organization (WHO)'s definition, which was part of the organization's constitution, adopted in 1946: "Health is a state of complete physical, mental and social well-being and not merely the absence of disease or infirmity" (WHO, 1948). In other words, being healthy is not just about not being sick but also about how you are thriving beyond the physical domain into the psychological and social aspects of your life. This fits quite nicely into the goals of health psychology and the framework of the biopsychosocial model.

Stephen King Gets Under My Skin

"Getting under the skin" is a phrase commonly used by health psychologists as an easy shorthand way of saying that a psychological or social experience has actually caused changes to the underlying structure of the human body. Just a very brief search of Google Scholar brings up several health psychology papers over the last few years that stress the adage. For example:

"Can poverty get under your skin? Basal cortisol levels and cognitive function in children from low and high socioeconomic status." (Lupien et al., 2001)
"How stress gets under the skin: cortisol and stress reactivity in psoriasis." (Evers et al., 2010)
"Under the skin: Using theories from biology and the social sciences to explore the mechanisms behind the black–white health gap." (Green et al., 2010)
"Brain on stress: how the social environment gets under the skin." (McEwen, 2012)
"Does attachment get under the skin? Adult romantic attachment and cortisol responses to stress." (Pietromonaco et al., 2013)
"How socioeconomic disadvantages get under the skin and into the brain to influence health development across the lifespan." (Kim et al., 2017)
"Getting under the skin: Children's health disparities as embodiment of social class." (Kramer et al., 2017)
"Getting under the skin: the association between social isolation and inflammatory markers." (Cudjoe et al., 2020)
"Getting under the skin: long-term links of adolescent peer relationship difficulties to adult vagal tone." (Allen et al., 2022)

And on and on and on. I suppose we can now add this book to the ever growing "Under the Skin" titles. But it is apt, as Stephen King really did get under my skin as I was reading *The Shining* alone in that hotel room. Simple words on a page had my heart racing like I was running a sprint and my body sweating like I had a high fever. How this happens, how it connects to health, and how we can use it to improve health are the focus of health psychology.

Health Psychology and *The Shining*

Just to give you a better and more specific view of what we are talking about in terms of health psychology, I want to give you a few examples of health psychology from *The Shining*. But first, just a quick aside. We cannot talk about any of this without first talking about the nervous system (see Figure 1.1). The nervous system is involved in all of our day-to-day activities. It includes our brain, our spinal cord, and all the nerves that extend out to the rest of our body. The brain and the spinal cord are called the central nervous system (CNS), and the peripheral nervous system (PNS) refers to those nerves that communicate with the rest of the body.

Let's start with the PNS, which itself is divided into the somatic nervous system and the autonomic nervous system (ANS). The somatic nervous system deals with activity that is voluntary – that is, we know the ways in which we want to move. For example, when Jack Torrence decides to pick up the roque mallet, he is using his somatic nervous system to send motor instructions from his CNS to the somatic periphery to make his muscles move.

As a whole, health psychology is not as interested in the somatic – getting under the skin implies something that is beyond the person's control. Thus, we spend much more time looking at the ANS. The ANS deals with involuntary actions – the

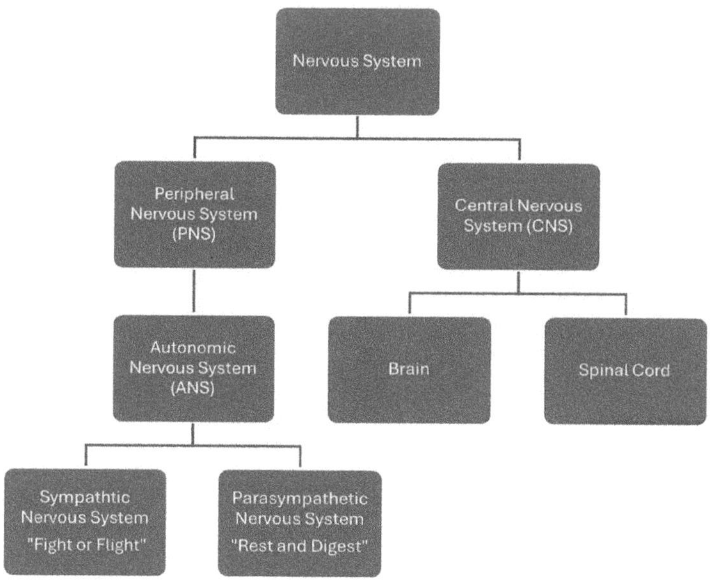

Figure 1.1 Divisions of the Nervous System within the Human Body.

things we have no control over – like the release of hormones from our glands or the movement of our heart muscles.

The actions of our ANS are divided into two main evolutionarily advantageous divisions – the sympathetic and the parasympathetic. The sympathetic division gets you ready for action – this is the "fight or flight" system, whereas the parasympathetic division helps you restore your systems – this would be the "rest and digest" system. For this book, since we are speaking of Stephen King, master of horror, we will mostly find ourselves in the land of the sympathetic nervous system.

Now, let's get back to CNS – specifically the brain. When first learning about the brain, it was very helpful for me to think about the "old" brain versus the "new" brain. The old brain includes the parts that are most like our animal counterparts, and these parts have been with us since the early days. It is responsible for all the things we need to survive – eating, sleeping, mating, fleeing, and fighting. This also includes basic emotions like fear, anger, and happiness. In essence, the old brain is simple but essential. Much of what is considered old brain is located in the lower parts of our brain – near the brain stem and underneath what you are probably picturing when you picture the human brain.

What most people imagine when they think of the human brain is the new brain – that is, the cerebral cortex (sometimes referred to as neocortex or new cortex). This is where the things that make us human are located – like complex problem solving, logical reasoning, and self-awareness. The cerebral cortex is divided into four main lobes – the frontal, parietal, temporal, and occipital (see Figure 1.2). The occipital is located at the back of the brain, and it mostly deals with visual processing. Parietal is concerned with touch and spatial processing, and the temporal is involved in auditory processing, language, and memory. The frontal lobe is of utmost importance when we talk about those things that make us human – what we call higher-level cognitive skills.

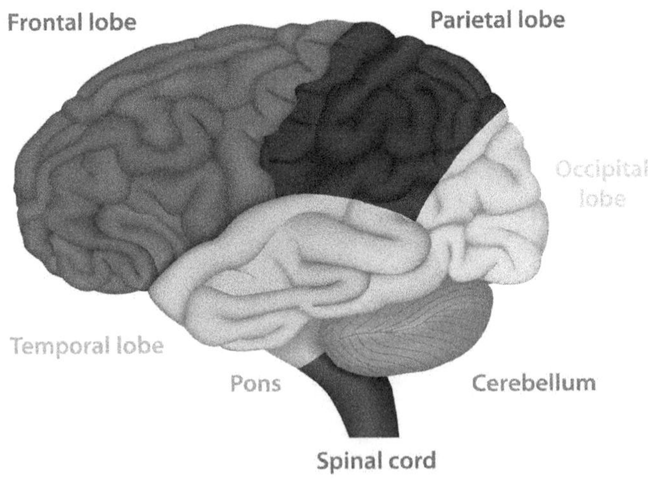

Figure 1.2 Main Lobes of the Human Brain.

But don't let this explanatory division fool you – these two "parts" of the brain have significant overlap and are in constant communication with each other and play key roles in what then gets sent to and received from the PNS and ANS. Throughout this book, you will get to know very specific parts of both the CNS and PNS, and we will begin now by using *The Shining* to demonstrate how some of it works.

Your Mouth Runs Dry

One biological mechanism that is intimately entwined with the health psychology concepts we will be talking about in this book is the hypothalamic-pituitary-adrenal (HPA) axis. It involves key brain structures of our CNS (hypothalamus, pituitary gland), and it then connects to the endocrine system via the ANS. This biological system is associated with our "fight or flight" reactions, and it was what *The Shining* was activating in my body while I read it in my Johnstown hotel room.

Figure 1.3 gives a good breakdown of what was happening while I was avoiding writing my dissertation by reading a book, including multiple "threats" hitting me at once. After some introspection, I think there were several psychological threats getting under my skin.

First, they don't let you stay in graduate school forever – you either leave with your PhD – your dissertation completed and defended – or you leave without it. I was very worried that my time was running out, and research has shown that impending deadlines are highly stressful and threatening (e.g., Sussman & Sekuler, 2022).

Second, I have always suffered from imposter syndrome – the feeling that you are not good enough for the current role you are pursuing. This constant self-doubt is extremely ego-threatening, and just like an impending deadline, it can be highly stressful and threatening (Chrousos et al., 2020).

Lastly, I think that Stephen King is just really good at creating a scene. And the scene he was creating in *The Shining* was so well-developed and illustrated, and so overlapping with my current situation, that my brain could not separate reality from fiction. I began to perceive threats where there were none. The fact that Jack Torrence is struggling to complete his play, as I was struggling to complete my dissertation, hit home. To finish it, he takes his family to a secluded hotel to diminish distractions, and yet is plagued with self-doubts, making the task much more difficult than he imagined. What was I thinking when I picked this book to read?

This created the perfect storm for my HPA axis to become activated. Reading the book, my brain was under siege. My hypothalamus interpreted several threats, and its solution was to get the body ready to fight or flee. A part of the hypothalamus known as the paraventricular nucleus then released corticotropin-releasing hormone (CRH), which traveled to the pituitary gland, which is located just underneath the hypothalamus. The CRH let the pituitary gland know something was up, and, in response, the pituitary released a hormone called adrenocorticotropic hormone (ACTH). The ACTH then traveled down through my blood to the top of my kidneys, where the adrenal cortex (the outer portion of the adrenal glands) is located. The adrenal cortex then produced cortisol (aka glucocorticoids), which is

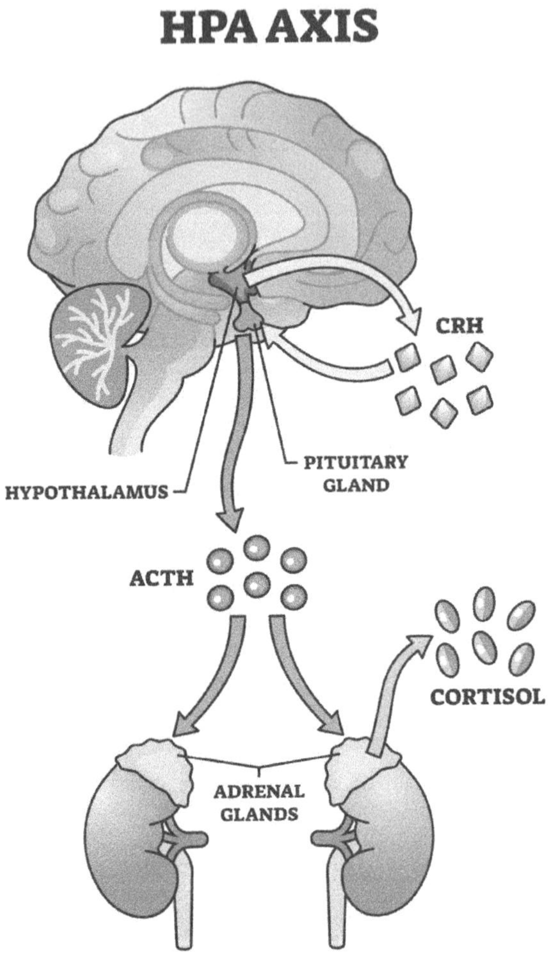

Figure 1.3 Hypothalamic-Pituitary-Adrenal (HPA) Axis Cascade.

known as the "stress hormone." All of these hormones released during this cascade have downstream effects on both our sympathetic and parasympathetic nervous systems that help us survive when faced with a fight or flight-style threat. In summary, what our minds perceive as threats in the world around us (whether real or imagined) are translated from psychological or social phenomena to the biological phenomena through the HPA axis.

While my own experiences illustrate this key biopsychosocial phenomenon, it is also painstakingly described by King himself in some of Jack Torrence's own experiences. In Chapter 23, "In the Playground," Jack ventures out on one of the last good days of fall to trim and prepare The Overlook's topiary animals for their long winter hibernation. It is here, while consciously understanding that the shrubbery rabbits, dogs, buffaloes, and lions are not real animals, his hypothalamus does begin the fight or flight response, maybe due to Jack's unconscious understanding of the evil nature of the hotel:

> Everything was just as it had been. So why had the flesh on his face and hands begun to creep, and why had the hair along the back of his neck begun to stand up, as if the flesh on his back had suddenly been tightened?
>
> (King, 2012, p.304)

What Jack is experiencing are some key aspects of the biology of the fight or flight response. When the cascade described above is instigated, the brain and body are trying to maximize survival. A threat has occurred, and in our most recent past as evolutionary creatures, that usual was a physical threat. The body needs to actually do something physical in order to stay safe. To ward off this threat, blood needs to flow to key areas – such as your lungs and heart, so that it can then send oxygenated blood to large muscles needed for physical exertion, such as running. In order to do this efficiently, it will start to reduce blood flow to the "non-essential" areas of the body – such as extremities. At the moment of great threat, you do not need blood to be flowing to your face or hands – and in this case, it resulted in those parts of Jack feeling numb or "creeping."

What is the deal with his hair standing up? This is probably also a result of sympathetic nervous system activation. What does your body do when you exert a lot of physical energy? You sweat to help keep your body from overheating. Part of this HPA axis cascade is activating your sweat glands in anticipation of the physical exertion of flighting or fleeing. When this happens, and the sweat starts, you basically become an electrical conduit (on a small scale!). The more stressed you are, the more your skin is able to conduct electricity, which leads to the possibility of the hair on your skin "standing up."

In health psychology, we use this as a way to measure sympathetic nervous system arousal – it is called a skin conductance test or galvanic skin response test. Study participants have electrodes placed on their fingers or hands, and the researchers administer a small and harmless electrical signal. The idea is that the more your skin conducts the signal, the more you experience sympathetic nervous system arousal.

Okay, let's get back to *The Shining*. Keep in mind that nothing actually threatening occurred to Jack, yet his mind and his fear made connections to his body, resulting in physiological changes. Here's health psychology![2] Jack experiences this again later in the book when he investigates the infamous Room 217, which has left Danny catatonic and the cook Dick Halloran swearing to never spend another season at The Overlook.

> A chilled finger pressed gently against the base of his spine, cooling him off ten degrees. It was joined by others, and they suddenly rippled all the way up his back to his medulla oblongata, playing his spine like a jungle instrument.

> His anger at Danny evaporated, and as he stepped forward and pushed the shower curtain back his mouth was dry and he felt only sympathy for his son and terror for himself.
>
> (King, 2012, p.371)

First let's talk about the obvious connection – the mention of the medulla oblongata. This is a part of the brain that is more commonly referred to as just the medulla. It is located right at the lower part of the brain stem, making it part of the old brain. The medulla is a key structure for a wide range of involuntary body functions – like breathing and heart functioning. It is also a key component in the brain connecting with the ANS – it is no wonder that Jack felt a physical "playing" of that part of his nervous system.

For the dry mouth aspect, we have to think back again to what the HPA axis is trying to do – save our lives by diverting resources to the systems that can help us meet our immediate fight or flight goals. One of the things that we don't need to be worrying about or spending energy on is digestion (remember, the opposite of fight or flight is "rest and digest"). Saliva production is a key part of our digestive process. It contains enzymes that immediately start to break down our food as soon as our teeth begin to physically break it down. As Jack faces the terror of whatever is in the bathtub of room 217, his nervous system has decided that digestion is not needed and has diverted resources away from saliva production. The result – Jack's mouth goes dry.

Box 1.3 The Epidemiologist's Bathtub

Room 217 of The Overlook Hotel is the room that Dick Halloran pleaded with Danny not to go into during the Torrences' overwinter stay. As Dick, and at least one of the chambermaids, knows, the room is haunted. More specifically, it is the bathroom that is haunted by the ghost of Lorraine Massey, a woman who died of a drug overdose in the bathtub. It is that bathroom and the bathtub that serve as a point of terror for both Danny and Jack Torrence.

Despite the horror of the Room 217 bathtub, there is a bathtub that you should familiarize yourself with in terms of health psychology. It is called the Epidemiologist's Bathtub (see Figure 1.4).

Throughout this book, we will be discussing some principles of epidemiology, the study of diseases – how, when, where, and among whom they show up. Since health psychology is concerned with the psychological, social, and biological factors of disease, epidemiology frameworks are constantly utilized. The most important ones are found in the epidemiologist's bathtub: morbidity, prevalence, incidence, and mortality. Morbidity is the number of cases of a specific disease or health outcome in a given group at a given time. There are two ways we can look at this: (1) the incidence, which is the number of new cases, and (2) the prevalence, which is the number of all new and existing cases within a given group at a given time. For example,

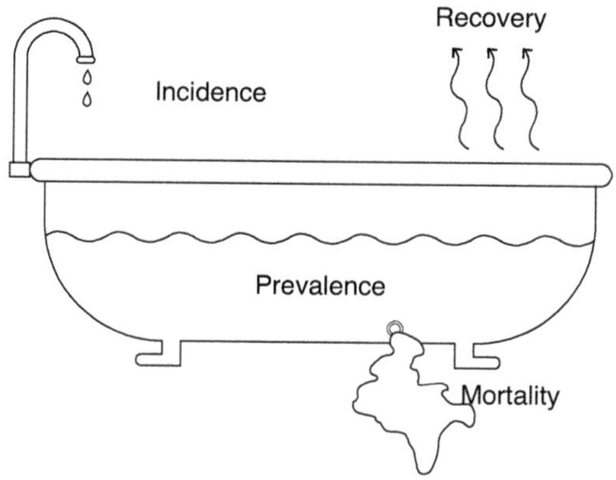

Figure 1.4 The Epidemiologist's Bathtub.

let's look at breast cancer among women in the United States (the given group) in 2022 (the given time).

Incidence: The number of new breast cancer cases in 2022 was 135.3 per 100,000 people.

Prevalence: The number of women living with breast cancer in the US in 2022 was 4,091,181.

Mortality is the number of people who die from a specific disease or outcome among a given group at a given time. In 2022, breast cancer mortality among US women was 18.9 per 100,000 people (National Cancer Institute, 2025).

Now take a look at the epidemiologist's bathtub again. The tub itself represents the given population at a given time concept we have been discussing. The water that is entering the tub represents the new cases or the incidence. The water already in the tub, along with the new water coming from the faucet, represents the prevalence (new and existing cases). The only way to leave the bathtub (no longer be considered a case) is either through dying (mortality; represented by the leak) or through recovery/cure (represented by evaporation).

Breaks Your Heart

> She had never dreamed there could be so much pain in life when there was nothing physically wrong. She hurt all the time.
>
> (King, 2012, p.72)

This, of course, is Wendy Torrence, thinking of her marriage to Jack, and the torment she felt when he was constantly deep in his cups with his coworker Al Shockley. What she is describing here is physical pain that results from emotional turmoil. Anyone who has had a "broken heart" knows exactly what we are talking about here.

The most obvious association here with health psychology is takotsubo cardiomyopathy (TCM), also known as broken heart syndrome (Peters et al., 2015). Cardiomyopathy is when the muscles of the heart change, either becoming larger, thicker, or more inflexible. This prevents the heart from pumping blood effectively and leads to chest pain. In TCM, the changes in the heart, and resulting heart pain, are most often caused by emotional stress, predominantly in women.

People who suffer from TCM do not have any significant coronary disease – they suffer from this as a result of things like death of a loved one or anniversary of death of a loved one, interpersonal conflict (Wendy felt pain when thinking about divorcing Jack), and intense moments of anxiety, anger, frustration, and fear (Sharkey et al., 2010). People have even experienced TCM in response to happy moments – getting married, becoming a grandparent, and winning at the casino (Ghadri et al., 2016).

This, of course, has led some to differentiate "broken heart syndrome" from "happy heart syndrome." Either way, what seems to be going on is that in reaction to experiencing an extreme emotion, the body is activating another one of those "fight or flight" reactions – this time not activating the HPA axis, but another axis called the sympatho-adreno-medullary (SAM) axis. It is very similar to the HPA axis, in that in response to the threat, or overwhelming emotion, the hypothalamus will release CRH, which will then induce the pituitary gland to secrete ACTH. However, from here, the ACTH goes to the adrenal medulla (as opposed to the adrenal cortex) and the adrenal medulla releases catecholamines, specifically epinephrine and norepinephrine (aka adrenaline and noradrenaline). Those with TCM have been found to have very high levels of catecholamines, and it is hypothesized that this surge in catecholamines may lead to changes in the cardiovascular system that result in TCM (Ono & Falcao, 2016).

Is this the pain that Wendy was referring to? It could be – but, of course, pain doesn't just have to occur in a specialized location in the heart. Wendy indicates that she hurts all the time, but she doesn't specify where. What she does discuss here is the loss of her father shortly after she marries Jack; she is thinking about losing Danny if she were to leave Jack and move in with her mother. She thinks about her mother rejecting her, about her own parents' divorce, and her impending one. The pain she may be describing here is social pain – the feelings we get when we experience loss, social rejection, and ostracism (Eisenberger, 2015).

Research on social pain, originally thought of as "just" a feeling, demonstrates that it may actually be physically painful. Wendy is indeed probably physically hurting. To understand why that might be, we have to return to this idea that what is going on in our bodies is evolutionarily adaptive – it is happening to help us survive. For humans, one of the key aspects of our lives that helps us in this pursuit is social connections. From the minute we are born, we rely on other people for our survival – we need someone to feed us, shelter us, clothe us, and comfort us. In the beginning, we cannot do this by ourselves, so making a bond with another human is essential. Our bodies may have adapted to make this bond more likely to occur and for us to be more apt to keep it going.

One way this may occur is through our opioid system, also known as our reward system. Activation of this system can result in feelings of happiness and pain relief. This is why opioid-based drugs can be so addictive – they trigger this system, providing the user with euphoria and pain reduction. The opioid system is a network that exists within the CNS and PNS. Within the brain, it is associated with old brain structures like the amygdala, which is the emotion center of the brain, and the mesolimbic pathway, which is key to reward and reinforcement. It also involves new brain structures like the prefrontal cortex, which is part of the frontal lobe, and the anterior cingulate cortex (ACC), which is involved in pain perception. Opioid receptors within the CNS can then inhibit pain messages received from the rest of the body through the PNS.

Evidence suggests that the body has actually adapted our opioid system to be sensitive to social connection and bonding. In essence, it is making sure we feel the "rewards" of being connected to another human being through increased feelings of happiness and reduction of physical pain. Thus, when we experience the rupture of our social connections, the opioid system will then warn us about this potential survival threat by having us experience pain (Eisenberger, 2015).

Throughout *The Shining*, we see Jack munching on aspirin to help with his headaches. If the social pain Wendy is experiencing is evolutionarily overlapping with physical pain, would it stand to reason that taking some aspirin would alleviate her pain as well? That is exactly the question that DeWall and colleagues (2010) asked in a fascinating study that compared a placebo to acetaminophen for reducing social pain.[3]

In a randomized controlled trial (RCT, see Box 1.4), the researchers randomly assigned 62 healthy undergraduates to receive either 500 mg of acetaminophen twice a day or the same dosage of placebo (an inactive substance). They did this every day for three weeks, and they also reported on their experience of "hurt feelings" resulting from social pain each day.

Box 1.4 Randomized Controlled Trials, the Gold Standard

The RCT is considered the gold standard in research. This is one of the best ways for researchers to see if something causes something else (in the example given in this chapter, does acetaminophen CAUSE the reduction of social pain?). We can get a much clearer sense of what is going on causally with this type of research because it addresses some key concepts.

By randomly assigning study participants to conditions – that is, subjects were randomly assigned to either get a placebo or acetaminophen – we reduce a lot of bias. That is, we can make sure that no particular group is over-represented in either group. If the assignment is truly random, we should have equal representation of age, sex, race, and so forth in each group.

Being controlled, it means that we have a comparison group, which is essential for figuring out whether the change is truly caused by the thing we are testing. If acetaminophen is truly what is reducing social pain, then we need to compare it to those not getting acetaminophen to show a true difference.

Another important aspect of these studies is that they are usually "double-blinded" – that is, neither the participant nor the researcher knows what the participant is receiving. They only know that they have either received the acetaminophen or the placebo. This helps control for expectancy effects – or changes in either the participants or the researcher's behavior because of what they expect will happen when given a certain treatment.

Be on the lookout for RCTs when researchers talk about causality, as that is the gold standard for investigating causal relationships.

What the researchers found was fascinating. At the beginning of the study, both the acetaminophen group and the placebo group had similar levels of hurt feelings. Those students taking the placebo pill daily showed no change in their level of hurt feelings throughout the three weeks. However, those students taking the acetaminophen experienced significant reductions in social pain/hurt feelings over the three weeks. So maybe she shouldn't be taking aspirin, but some Tylenol might be just what Wendy needs (and perhaps something a bit stronger after the ordeal at The Overlook ends)!

Takes Your Breath Away

> For Wendy, it was like discovering truth in a cliche: her breath was taken away. For a moment she was unable to breath at all; the view had knocked the wind out of her.
>
> (King, 2012, p.89)

Who hasn't experienced having their breath taken away? For Wendy Torrence, it occurs when she first looks out through the peaks of the Colorado mountains to see The Overlook for the first time. Her breath is taken away by a combination of feelings – wonderment at the beauty of the place and fear of the height at which they stand. Is what she feels true – can our minds really take control of our respiratory system?

The respiratory system is, of course, the group of organs and biological structures that allow us to breathe. We need to breathe in oxygen-rich air to supply our body with the energy it needs to function, and we need to breathe out the carbon dioxide-rich byproduct. Obviously, breathing is key to our survival and always has been – so the part of the CNS that controls breathing is located in the old brain – the medulla in the brain stem and another structure just above it called the pons.

Respiration is an important aspect of ANS activation. When your sympathetic nervous system prepares your body for action, it needs to get in as much oxygen-rich blood as possible. The medulla and pons will speed up your breathing, the airways in your lungs will open up to let more air flow in, and mucus production will decrease, so there is not as much substance blocking different airways. As we have discussed before, the sympathetic nervous system is triggered by your perception of threats, and strong emotions are indicative of threat. This may be why the extreme emotion of wonderment, along with fear of the height, causes Wendy to have difficulty breathing – the quick increase of her rate of breathing may have taken her by surprise.

We actually know quite a lot about the mind-respiratory system connection due to one disease – asthma. Asthma is an old disease – written records of the disease go as far back as ancient Greece and Rome (Jackson, 2009). It is an illness that causes the airways to narrow, resulting in shortness of breath and the characteristic wheeze. It is one of the "Holy Seven" of psychosomatic disease – those illnesses in which psychological states contribute to symptoms (Dunbar, 1947; see Box 2.4 in Chapter 2 for a full list). We will talk a lot more about this when we talk about *It*, Eddie Kaspbrak, and the placebo effect. The important takeaway here is that asthma, and the respiratory system by association, has always been a key player in health psychology. And how does asthma connect to *The Shining*? Check out Box 1.5 for a fascinating history of how childhood asthma was once treated in the state of Colorado.

Box 1.5 The Stanley Hotel, Colorado Air, and the Parentectomy

One of the main characters in *The Shining* is actually the Overlook Hotel, which haunts Jack Torrence and his family throughout their short time as winter hotel caretakers. The model for The Overlook is The Stanley Hotel in Estes Park, Colorado (Figure 1.5). The Stanley Hotel was built by Freelan Oscar Stanley, known for inventing a steam-powered automobile. In the early 1900s, Stanley traveled to Colorado and the Rocky Mountains to help relieve a recurrence of tuberculosis, a bacterial infection that mostly affects the lungs. At the time, many people felt the air within the mountains had curative properties, especially for lung disorders. Indeed, Stanley did get better and attributed his improvement to the mountain air and decided to build a house in Estes Park, and later a hotel, so others could enjoy the rest, relaxation, and health restoration the mountains provided him.

Of course, tuberculosis is not the only lung disease that has shown improvement in the setting of *The Shining*. About 65 miles from Estes Park is Denver, where in the 1940s, an allergist named M. Murray Peshkin was treating children with asthma with a procedure known as a "parentectomy." The procedure involved the removal of children with "intractable" asthma from their parents for long periods of time. Intractable means that the children's asthma was not getting better, even with the most modern of medications and treatments available. Peshkin was very invested in the idea that for those children whose asthma was resistant to treatment, their asthma was more somatic – sensitive to anxiety and conflict and psychological factors

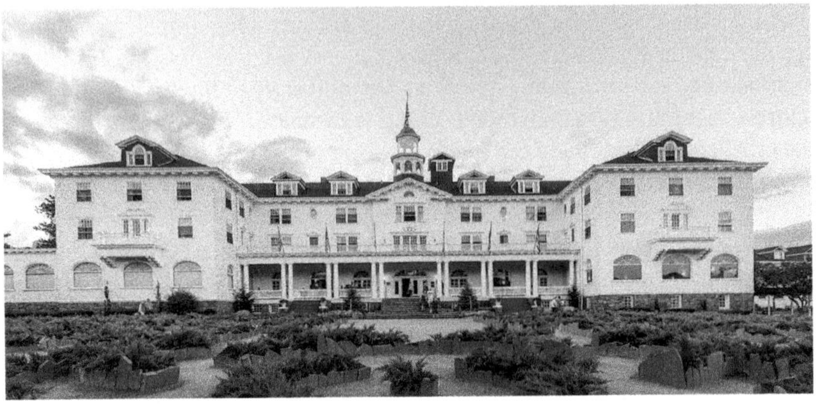

Figure 1.5 The Stanley Hotel.

(Peshkin, 1966). According to Peshkin, about 10% of children with asthma had a more "psychogenic" variation of asthma (Peshkin, 1964), and thus, the treatment must be more psychosocial in nature.

At this time, many medical professionals believed that this psychological conflict among children with asthma was coming from their parents, particularly their mothers (Gervais, 1966). It was proposed that separating children from their parents is what was needed to see improvement in their asthma, hence the parentectomy. Yet where are these children supposed to go? Now here is where the Stanley Hotel comes into the picture. Remember, the Stanley Hotel was used as a health retreat for those with tuberculosis. The high rate of tuberculosis patients in Colorado also meant that there was an increase in children who lost their parents, either for just the time they were in treatment or because the parents succumbed to the illness. Recognizing that these orphaned children needed care, a group of women started the Denver Sheltering Home for Jewish Children. When tuberculosis was no longer the threat it once was, the Sheltering Home became the location where those children with asthma could live out of the reach of their parents. It became the Children's Asthma Research Institute and Hospital (Hughes, 2021).

Children aged 5–15 years were separated from their parents for 18–24 months (with visits allowed every 6 months), and Peshkin claimed that 99% of the children showed significant improvement or were completely free of their asthma by the end. So why aren't parentectomies done today if the success rate was so high? For the most part, it almost seems like a plot worthy of King – young children taken away from their parents for years during key developmental periods. Many felt that the potential harm that could occur from family separation far outweighed the benefits, especially as asthma treatment improved (Pinkerton et al., 1971), and eventually, it fell out of vogue.

Turns Your Stomach

> And so he had hung up, and that was when the cramps had come, hitting him like lightning bolts, making him curl up in front of the telephone like a penitent, hands over his belly, head throbbing like a monstrous bladder.
>
> (King, 2012, p.279)

What is described above happens immediately after Jack gets off the phone with Al Shockley, Jack's old drinking buddy, and the man who got him the job at The Overlook. They have just had a heated conversation in which Al exerts his dominance over Jack and tells him he is not to write a book about The Overlook, an idea which has lately been dominating Jack's mind. When told this, Jack immediately is filled with rage, though he hides it from Al. However, after the interaction, he is crippled by intense abdominal cramps.

What happened to Jack? Was it something he ate? As you can probably guess, it was not any food that he ate, but the anger he had to swallow. The intense emotional reaction to Al's admonishments probably activated another nervous system that we have yet to discuss – the enteric nervous system (ENS). Amazingly, there are more neurons in your gastrointestinal tract than in your spinal cord (Purves et al., 2004, p. 479). Your CNS is able to communicate with the ENS through what we refer to as the gut–brain axis. More recently, we have moved to an understanding that the gut–brain axis doesn't just consist of the brain and gut, but that it also includes our microbiome (Mayer et al., 2022). The microbiome consists of all the microorganisms that live within us, and most of these reside within our digestive system. The idea is that the brain, the ENS, and our microbiome are in constant communication with each other. The question is, what might have been communicated when Jack ended his phone call with Al?

We know that the gut–brain–microbiome axis is heavily connected to the ANS and the HPA axis. Jack was definitely experiencing Al's ultimatum as a threat, and as such, his fight or flight response was activated. What is not essential when fighting or fleeing? Digestion. Thus, the CNS may communicate to the ENS to stop what it is doing – that is, it interrupts gut motility, which is basically the movement of food through your digestive tract. This could definitely lead to the pain and discomfort that Jack suddenly feels.

Jack has one other thing working against him when it comes to his psychological distress turning into gut cramps – his history of alcohol use. Alcohol use has been associated with changes in the makeup and functioning of the microbiome (Leclercq et al., 2014). This could have the potential for making Jack's gut–brain axis more sensitive to stress signals from the CNS, or it could be working in multiple directions. Carbia and colleagues (2021) have discussed a complicated "loop" effect, where alcohol impacts the microbiome, which then communicates with the CNS in such a way that emotional processing becomes difficult, which then may make alcohol more likely to be used by the stressed individual. This is really fascinating new science, and it highlights the latest in health psychology research. However, people, like Jack, have been feeling these effects for centuries.

Laughter Is the Best Medicine

In this introductory chapter, I have spent an inordinate amount of time describing the negative health outcomes in health psychology and the biopsychosocial model. Yet there is plenty of research showing the benefits of our psychological and social worlds on our biology and longevity. It is just a bit harder to find examples of this in Stephen King's world!

However, I did find one, and it is a great scene that occurs when Jack, Wendy, and Danny first arrive at The Overlook. During the hustle and bustle of the last day of full operations for the hotel, as people are checking out, and the last preparations for the closing are made, Wendy sits and people-watches. Her eye gazes toward the huge fireplace alit in the lobby, and she notices three nuns:

> Three nuns sat on a sofa that was drawn up almost to the hearth itself. They were talking and smiling with their bags stacked up on either side, waiting for the checkout line to thin a little. As Wendy watched them, they burst into a chord of tinkly, girlish laughter. She felt a smile touch her own lips; not one of them could be under sixty.
>
> (King, 2012, p.92)

This scene in the book brings to mind three important concepts in health psychology: aging, happiness, and nuns. Why nuns? Well, in health psychology, there is a fairly famous research project known as "The Nun Study." The Nun Study was what we call a longitudinal study – that is, it followed the participants over time and collected data in intervals throughout the study period. Data collection began in 1991, and the participants were 678 Catholic nuns who were part of the same congregation (Clarke et al., 2024). At the beginning of the study, they ranged in age between 75 and 102 years old. Nuns are unique in that most of them join their congregations early, and as such live lives that are very similar to one another – they live in the same types of homes, and they have the same income, food, healthcare, marital status, parent status, and social networks. In this way, we can look for ways in which they are different that may have an impact on their health and well-being.[4]

The Nun Study collected a lot of interesting data. In addition to having years of medical and dental records, they also had autobiographies that the nuns had written as young women joining the congregation. Additionally, the nuns went through intense neuropsychological assessments – the main purpose being to detect dementia as they aged (Snowdon, 2003). The Nun Study went on for decades, and so, it was able to study the morbidity and mortality (see Box 1.3) of the nuns.

What this scene in *The Shining* reminded me of was the study published by the researchers in 2001 (Danner et al.). They went back and analyzed the nun's autobiographies – they coded them for the number of words that they used that indicate positive emotion (happiness, love, hope, etc.), negative emotion (sadness, fear, shame, etc.), and neutral emotion (surprise). They then looked at the mortality rates among the nuns – who had died and who were still living at the time of the data analysis. What they found was that the more positive words a nun used in her autobiography, the more likely she was to be alive. Looking at those who used the least amount of positive emotion words to those who used the most, there was a 2.5-fold increase in death among the low positive words group. Happier nuns live longer lives! Chances are those laughing nuns at The Overlook have a long life ahead of them (unlike some of the Torrences).

This relationship between positive emotions and health and longevity continues to be an important aspect of health psychology, and the evidence for the link has grown substantially since this finding (Pressman et al., 2019). Despite the use of Stephen King's works as a means for explanation, I will try to find as many non-scary examples like this throughout the book – if only so that the positive emotions you feel can make you a wee bit healthier!

Is It Under Your Skin Yet?

Has health psychology gotten under your skin yet? If not, don't worry, it will!

While my experience of *The Shining* at the Holiday Inn was terrifying, it was also exhilarating. I was fully invested in Jack, Wendy, and Danny, and the story King told. This started my King journey, which has ultimately led to this book. With every novel or short story of King's that I read – the connections with my own discipline and expertise manifested themselves. The overlap of what was going on in places like Castle Rock, Derry, and Boulder's Free Zone and what I was teaching and researching was constantly present.

I hope that this introduction gives you a good taste of what health psychology is and what is to come. This book will further explore the mind–body connections present in King's work, in hopes of further explaining the basic foundations and concepts that direct the field of health psychology. Chapter 2 will delve a bit deeper into the history of health psychology and how it got to where it is now, and it will do the same thing with Stephen King. In Chapter 3, we will use *Pet Sematary* and *The Dark Half* to illustrate the research methods and approaches that are key to studying health psychology. The miraculous power of the placebo effect, a continuous theme throughout many of King's works, will be introduced in Chapter 4, specifically looking at *Thinner*, *It*, and *Holly*. Bill Hodges, of *The Bill Hodges Trilogy,* will guide us through an exploration of how occupation, retirement, and other individual aspects of our lives impact our health in Chapter 5. Chapter 6 will explore the world of *The Running Man* to explain the impact of socioeconomic status and larger macro-level influences on our health. Adverse childhood experiences and their detrimental influence on health in later life will be the topic discussed through the characters in *The Body* in Chapter 7. Through King's epic *The Stand,* Chapter 8 will explore infectious disease and how the immune system is responsive to the psychological and social factors we are exposed to every day. What exactly sleep is, how it impacts our health, and the role of aging will be the focus of Chapter 9, which takes place in the Derry of *Insomnia*. Lastly, Chapter 10 will talk about one of the scariest topics of all – actually changing our behaviors to better our health – through the short story *Quitters, Inc.*

I hope that you will be able to be a better person than my younger self, put any preconceived notions of who Stephen King is and what he writes aside, so that we can go on this adventure together, exploring how his stories really can get under your skin.

Versions of *The Shining*

Novel: King, S. (1977). *The Shining*. Doubleday.

Novel: Kindle Edition (Where quotes are from): King, S. (2012). *The Shining*. Random House. https://www.amazon.com/dp/B0078XGJXO

Film: Kubrick, S. (Director). (1980). *The Shining* [Film]. Warner Bros.

TV Miniseries: Garris, M. (Director). (1997). *Stephen King's* The Shining [TV miniseries]. Warner Bros Television.

Audiobook (Audible Edition): King, S. (2012). *The Shining* (C. Scott, Narr.) [Audiobook]. Random House Audio. https://www.audible.com/pd/The-Shining-Audiobook/B008OLF29Q[5]

Learn More Questions

1 We discussed threats and stressors as being a main component of getting the biological systems to begin the work of flight or fight. Can you see other examples throughout *The Shining* where these mechanisms are occurring? Provide an example from the book and then explain what might be going on in the characters' body based on what you learned in this chapter.

2 Jack Torrence suffers from alcohol abuse disorder (AUD). Look up the *Diagnostic and Statistical Manual of Mental Disorders* (DSM) 5 criteria for AUD. What criteria does Jack meet? Provide specific examples. Based on what you have learned in this chapter, what role do you think the opioid system might play in Jack's alcohol use?

Notes

1 The story of the Johnstown Flood is fascinating, and you should check out David McCullough's masterful book about the topic: McCullough, D. (1968). *The Johnstown flood: The incredible story behind one of the most devastating disasters America has ever known*. Simon & Schuster.

2 My apologies to Stephen King, as this is a reference to Stanley Kubrik's 1980 film adaptation of *The Shining*, of which King is purportedly not a fan.

3 We will discuss placebos (and nocebos) in great detail in Chapter 4.

4 We refer to this as individual differences, and this will be discussed more in Chapter 5.

5 I think Campbell Scott does an absolutely fantastic job reading *The Shining* here. As a Gen X'er, I am a bit biased, as I had a huge teenage crush on him (I'm still crying from *Dying Young*), but still, I highly recommend.

Bibliography

Allen, J. P., Loeb, E. L., Davis, A. A., Costello, M. A., & Uchino, B. N. (2022). Getting under the skin: Long-term links of adolescent peer relationship difficulties to adult vagal tone. *Journal of Behavioral Medicine, 45*(5), 690–701. https://doi.org/10.1007/s10865-022-00334-1

Bentley, J. (1975). Some thoughts on parentectomy. *Journal of Asthma Research, 12*(3), 125–128. https://doi.org/10.3109/02770907509098941

Carbia, C., Lannoy, S., Maurage, P., López-Caneda, E., O'Riordan, K. J., Dinan, T. G., & Cryan, J. F. (2021). A biological framework for emotional dysregulation in alcohol misuse: From gut to brain. *Molecular Psychiatry, 26*(4), 1098–1118.

Chrousos, G. P., Mentis, A. F. A., & Dardiotis, E. (2020). Focusing on the neuro-psychobiological and evolutionary underpinnings of the imposter syndrome. *Frontiers in Psychology, 11*, 1553. https://doi.org/10.3389/fpsyg.2020.01553

Clarke, K. M., Etemadmoghadam, S., Danner, B., Corbett, C., Ghaseminejad-Bandpey, A., Dopler, M., … & Flanagan, M. E. (2025). The nun study: Insights from 30 years of aging and dementia research. *Alzheimer's & Dementia, 21*(2), e14626. https://doi.org/10.1002/alz.14626

Cudjoe, T. K., Latkin, C., Roth, D., Thorpe Jr, R., & Boyd, C. (2020). Getting under the skin: The association between social isolation and inflammatory markers. *Innovation in Aging, 4*(Suppl 1), 589. https://doi.org/10.1093/geroni/igaa057.1975

Danner, D. D., Snowdon, D. A., & Friesen, W. V. (2001). Positive emotions in early life and longevity: Findings from the nun study. *Journal of Personality and Social Psychology, 80*(5), 804. https://doi.org/10.1037/0022-3514.80.5.804

DeWall, C. N., MacDonald, G., Webster, G. D., Masten, C. L., Baumeister, R. F., Powell, C., … & Eisenberger, N. I. (2010). Acetaminophen reduces social pain: Behavioral and neural evidence. *Psychological Science, 21*(7), 931–937. https://doi.org/10.1177/0956797610374741/

Dunbar, H. F. (1947). *Mind and body: Psychosomatic medicine*. Random House.

Eisenberger, N. I. (2015). Social pain and the brain: Controversies, questions, and where to go from here. *Annual Review of Psychology, 66*(1), 601–629. https://doi.org/10.1146/annurev-psych-010213-115146

Evers, A. W. M., Verhoeven, E. W. M., Kraaimaat, F. W., De Jong, E. M. G. J., De Brouwer, S. J. M., Schalkwijk, J., … & Van De Kerkhof, P. C. M. (2010). How stress gets under the skin: Cortisol and stress reactivity in psoriasis. *British Journal of Dermatology, 163*(5), 986–991. https://doi.org/10.1111/j.1365-2133.2010.09984.x

Gervais, L. (1966). Bronchial asthma and identification with the aggressor. *Canadian Psychiatric Association Journal, 11*(6), 497–500. https://doi.org/10.1177/070674376601100607

Ghadri, J. R., Sarcon, A., Diekmann, J., Bataiosu, D. R., Cammann, V. L., Jurisic, S., … & Prasad, A. (2016). Happy heart syndrome: Role of positive emotional stress in takotsubo syndrome. *European Heart Journal, 37*(37), 2823–2829. https://doi.org/10.1093/eurheartj/ehv757

Green, T. L., & Darity Jr, W. A. (2010). Under the skin: Using theories from biology and the social sciences to explore the mechanisms behind the black–white health gap. *American Journal of Public Health, 100*(S1), S36–S40. https://doi.org/10.2105/AJPH.2009.171140

Hughes, H. L. (2021, March 19). *The untold stories of the Denver hospital that pioneered "parentectomy"—and saved children's lives*. 5280. https://www.5280.com/the-untold-stories-of-the-denver-hospital-that-pioneered-parentectomy-and-saved-childrens-lives/

Jackson, M. (2009). *Asthma: The biography*. Oxford University Press. https://doi.org/10.1093/oso/9780199237951.001.0001

Kim, P., Evans, G. W., Chen, E., Miller, G., Seeman, T. (2018). How socioeconomic disadvantages get under the skin and into the brain to influence health development across the lifespan. In: Halfon, N., Forrest, C., Lerner, R., Faustman, E. (eds.), *Handbook of Life Course Health Development*. Springer, Cham. https://doi.org/10.1007/978-3-319-47143-3_19

King, S. (2012). *The Shining*. Random House. https://www.amazon.com/dp/B0078XGJXO

Kramer, M. R., Schneider, E. B., Kane, J. B., Margerison-Zilko, C., Jones-Smith, J., King, K., … & Grzywacz, J. G. (2017). Getting under the skin: Children's health disparities as embodiment of social class. *Population Research and Policy Review, 36*(5), 671–697. https://doi.org/10.1007/s11113-017-9431-7

Lacey, C., Mulder, R., Bridgman, P., Kimber, B., Zarifeh, J., Kennedy, M., & Cameron, V. (2014). Broken heart syndrome—Is it a psychosomatic disorder? *Journal of Psychosomatic Research, 77*(2), 158–160. https://doi.org/10.1016/j.jpsychores.2014.05.003

Leclercq, S., Matamoros, S., Cani, P. D., Neyrinck, A. M., Jamar, F., Stärkel, P., … & Delzenne, N. M. (2014). Intestinal permeability, gut-bacterial dysbiosis, and behavioral markers of alcohol-dependence severity. *Proceedings of the National Academy of Sciences, 111*(42), E4485–E4493. https://doi.org/10.1073/pnas.1415174111

Lupien, S. J., King, S., Meaney, M. J., & McEwen, B. S. (2001). Can poverty get under your skin? Basal cortisol levels and cognitive function in children from low and high socioeconomic status. *Development and Psychopathology, 13*(3), 653–676. https://doi.org/10.1017/S0954579401003133

Mayer, E. A., Nance, K., & Chen, S. (2022). The gut–brain axis. *Annual Review of Medicine, 73*(1), 439–453. https://doi.org/10.1146/annurev-med-042320-014032

McEwen, B. S. (2012). Brain on stress: How the social environment gets under the skin. *Proceedings of the National Academy of Sciences, 109*(supplement_2), 17180–17185. https://doi.org/10.1073/pnas.1121254109

National Cancer Institute. (2025). *Cancer stat facts: Female breast cancer*. Surveillance, Epidemiology, and End Results Program. https://seer.cancer.gov/statfacts/html/breast.html

Ono, R., & Falcão, L. M. (2016). Takotsubo cardiomyopathy systematic review: Pathophysiologic process, clinical presentation and diagnostic approach to Takotsubo cardiomyopathy. *International Journal of Cardiology, 209*, 196–205. https://doi.org/10.1016/j.ijcard.2016.02.012

Peshkin, M. (1959). Intractable asthma of childhood rehabilitation at the institutional level with a follow-up of 150 cases. *International Archives of Allergy and Immunology, 15*(1–3), 91–112. https://doi.org/10.1159/000229036

Peshkin, M. M. (1964). The role of the non-psychiatrist in psychosomatic medicine. *Psychosomatics 5*(6), 335–340.

Peshkin, M. M. (1966). The responsibility of the convalescent asthma home, the physician, and the community to the intractably asthmatic child. *Journal of Asthma Research, 4*(1), 13–17. https://doi.org/10.3109/02770906609100301

Peters, M. N., George, P., & Irimpen, A. M. (2015). The broken heart syndrome: Takotsubo cardiomyopathy. *Trends in Cardiovascular Medicine, 25*(4), 351–357. https://doi.org/10.1016/j.tcm.2014.11.005

Pietromonaco, P. R., DeBuse, C. J., & Powers, S. I. (2013). Does attachment get under the skin? Adult romantic attachment and cortisol responses to stress. *Current Directions in Psychological Science, 22*(1), 63–68. https://doi.org/10.1177/0963721412463229

Pinkerton, P., Weaver, C. M., & Henry, K. (1971). Reappraisal of "parentectomy" in childhood asthma. *Medical Officer, 125*(5), 63–65.

Pressman, S. D., Jenkins, B. N., & Moskowitz, J. T. (2019). Positive affect and health: What do we know and where next should we go? *Annual Review of Psychology, 70*(1), 627–650. https://doi.org/10.1146/annurev-psych-010418-102955

Purves, D., Augustine, G. J., Fitzpatrick, D., Hall, W. C., LaMantia, A.-S., McNamara, J. O., & White, L. E. (2004). *Neuroscience*. (3rd ed.). Sinauer Associates.

Sharkey, S. W., Windenburg, D. C., Lesser, J. R., Maron, M. S., Hauser, R. G., Lesser, J. N., … & Maron, B. J. (2010). Natural history and expansive clinical profile of stress (tako-tsubo) cardiomyopathy. *Journal of the American College of Cardiology, 55*(4), 333–341. https://doi.org/10.1016/j.jacc.2009.08.057

Snowdon, D. A. (2003). Healthy aging and dementia: Findings from the Nun Study. *Annals of Internal Medicine, 139*(5_Part_2), 450–454. https://doi.org/10.7326/0003-4819-139-5_part_2-200309021-00014

Sussman, R. F., & Sekuler, R. (2022). Feeling rushed? Perceived time pressure impacts executive function and stress. *Acta Psychologica, 229*, 103702. https://doi.org/10.1016/j.actpsy.2022.103702

World Health Organization. (1948). Summary reports on proceedings minutes and final acts of the international health conference held in New York from 19 June to 22 July 1946. New York: WHO, 35.

2 Beginnings

The History of Health Psychology and Stephen King

Introduction

In this chapter, we will explore both how Stephen King developed into the author he is today and health psychology became the field it is today. On paper, Stephen King, born in 1947, is technically older than health psychology, which was officially recognized as a psychology subfield by the American Psychological Association in 1978. However, at its core, health psychology has been around since the time of the earliest civilizations. Of course, Stephen King hasn't been around since the dawn of human time, but the themes in which he works certainly have. And as is the point of this book, I hope to point out how these long-present health psychology concepts, and the developed themes of Stephen King, overlap.

We have already talked a bit in Chapter 1 about what health psychology is. Before we move on to its history, though, let's explore who Stephen King is and why health psychology may play a role in his writing, whether consciously or unconsciously.

The Start of Stephen King

Stephen King was born in the state of Maine on September 21st, 1947. At his birth, his family was made up of his older brother David, his mother Ruth, and his father Donald. However, Donald left the family when King was around two years old and was not seen again. Following work and family when times were hard, King and his mother and brother moved around the US – living in Maine, Wisconsin, Indiana, and Connecticut. While King states that his childhood was ordinary, in Chapter 7, we will discuss adverse childhood experiences (ACEs), of which King experienced many. From the loss of his father at an early age, to the constant moving of home, to the lower economic status of his single-parent home, he may have experienced some manifestations of health psychology throughout his life.

For example, physical health-wise, King has described several harrowing childhood experiences revolving around doctors' visits. Probably the most ingrained in my mind is the story King tells in his book *On Writing: A Memoir of the Craft*. King describes spending most of the first grade at home, sick with the measles, strep throat, high fevers, and very painful ears. Unfortunately, during this time, he had

DOI: 10.4324/9781003495994-2

three interactions with a needle-happy doctor who pierced his eardrums each time, which was on equal footing in terms of pain with him infamously getting hit by a car in 1999 (to be discussed later in this chapter). To this day, King describes the smell of rubbing alcohol as a trigger for those traumatic childhood medical experiences.

What causes those painful early life experiences were infectious viruses and bacteria, and we will talk more about how King's early life experiences may have made him more susceptible. We will explore how one section of health psychology branched off into psychoneuroimmunology – the study of how psychological factors interplay with your nervous system, ultimately leading to changes to the immune system (Chapter 8, looking at *The Stand*, will tackle this in-depth). Eventually, when he was around six, he had to have his tonsils removed, and he started the first grade over again when he was well again the next year. It was during this bed-bound year that he began exploring comic books and stories, which eventually led to his own early experiments with storytelling. As much as that year of medical challenges may have impacted King, we may feel lucky that it created the time for him to explore tale-telling at such an early age.

As King was growing up in the 1950s and 1960s, some key things were happening in the field of psychology that began the development of health psychology into its own discipline. But before we get there, it may be apt for us to go WAY, WAY, WAY back and discuss some of the history of the idea of thinking about the mind and body (psychology and biology) as being intimately entwined. While the biomedical model (see Box 2.1) dominated much of the 20th century, and some may argue it still does today, this wasn't always the case.

Box 2.1 The Biomedical Model

When Stephen King was born in 1947, the approach to health in the United States was deeply entrenched in the biomedical model. What exactly is the biomedical model? It is the idea that health and illness are derived solely from biological factors. It is one of the defining characteristics of Western medicine (as opposed to Eastern traditions, which are seen as more holistic). Amazingly enough, the foundations of our current biomedical model started in the 1600s, with the development of the earliest microscopes. These microscopes allowed us to explore cells and bacteria and identify specific pathogens linked to disease. Thus, germ theory was developed – the idea that most of the diseases that humans suffer from (at least at the time) stem from the various microorganisms that were seen under the microscope.

Germ theory and the biomedical model have guided medical treatment in the United States ever since. However, as we will discuss, something occurred in the 20th century that has caused a shift in how we approach health and illness – the epidemiological transition. The epidemiological transition refers to the changes that occurred in the leading causes of death in the 20th century, as well as life expectancy. Figure 2.1 shows the life expectancy in years from 1880 to 2023 – there was a significant increase from life expectancies of 40 or 50 years, to well into the 70s or 80s a hundred years later.[1]

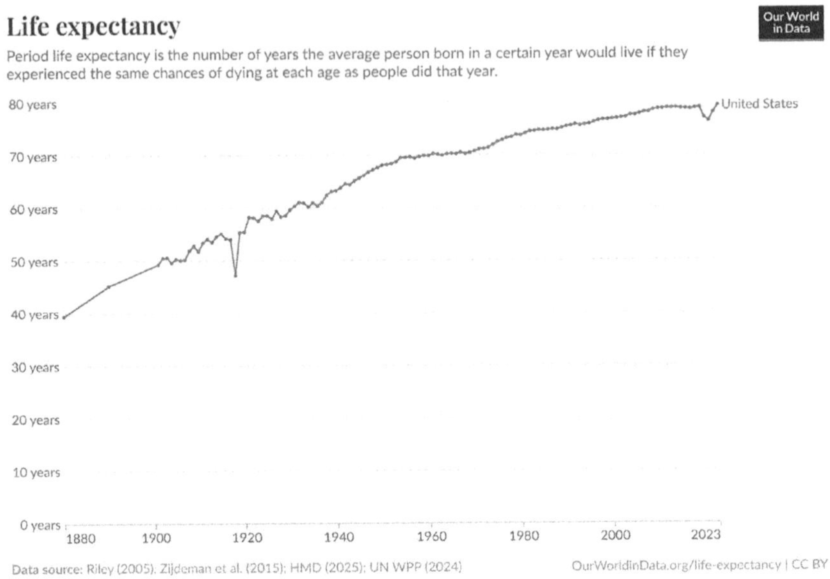

Figure 2.1 Life Expectancy in Years 1880– 2023.

Why the shift? Well, we can thank the biomedical model for that. Focusing on germs, pathogens, and bacteria meant we developed better sanitation methods, better food treatments and storage, vaccines, and medications that significantly reduced the impact of communicable diseases. What it shifted into was the rise of non-communicable diseases – or diseases of lifestyle – such as diabetes, cancer, and cardiovascular disease. The biomedical model hasn't been as effective at tackling these health problems, which has led to a shift – occurring throughout Stephen King's lifetime – to the biopsychosocial model, which is the focus of this book.

The Start of Health Psychology

The Mind–Body Debate

Throughout much of the written history, and probably before, there has been a great debate about whether or not we should consider the mind and body as two distinct entities. In ancient times, Plato believed that the mind and body were separate, with your mind living on even when your body dies. Aristotle, as well as other Greeks like Galen, saw mind and body as being integrated. Most famously, in the 17th century, we had Descartes, who pursued dualism, the idea that the mind and body are distinct. This Descartes dualism is important when we consider what else was going on in the 17th, 18th, and 19th centuries in terms of the biomedical model.

Much like Descartes, the "modern" medicine of these times held that one could treat the body as a separate entity from the mind, and that was the guiding position of most physicians and scientists of the time. As we will discuss, though, this began to change in the mid-20th century, and it led to the advent of the fields of psychosomatic medicine and health psychology in the latter parts of the century.

Importantly for us here, I think the evidence will show that Stephen King is not a dualist, and he fully believes that body and mind are entwined, as well as our awareness and interactions beyond our own worlds, bodies, and thoughts. Let us then explore how these ideas developed, in both the health psychology arena and within the life and works of Stephen King.

Trephination – Like Something Out of a Stephen King Novel

Health psychology is often discussed as the study of the connection between mind and body. The idea that the thing that is located on the top of our neck and shoulders has an important role to play in what goes on in the rest of our body is a concept that can be shown to have been in existence among our earliest ancestors. Archeologists have uncovered skulls of people of prehistoric cultures that show evidence

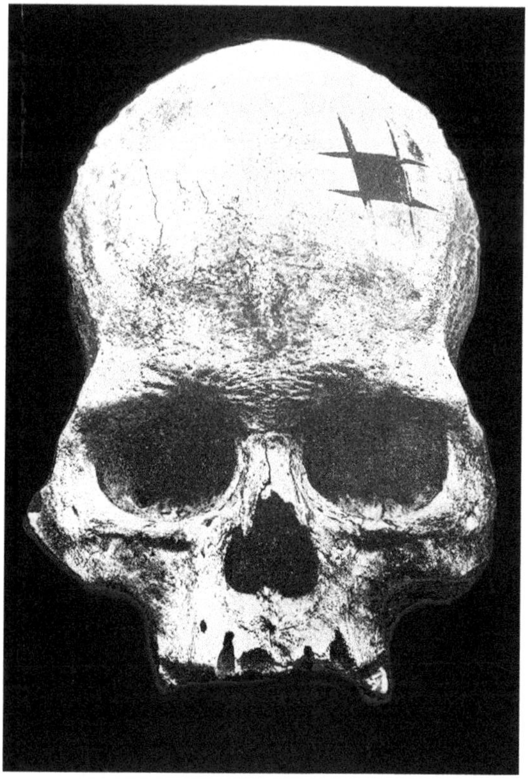

Figure 2.2 Trephined Skull.

of trephination – a procedure in which a part of the human skull is removed in order to treat various illnesses and disabilities (Nanayakkara & Gunarathne, 2022).

Basically, drilling a hole into the skull (though it probably wasn't a drill, as evidenced by the hack marks on the skull in Figure 2.2), ancient practitioners thought that they would be curing a wide range of maladies, mostly caused by evil spirits that lived in the brain that must be released. Nothing sounds more Stephen King than that!

The Humors of Ancient Greece

Trephination techniques for healing the physical health of individuals continued along until Ancient Greece, where it was still being used, but more so for actually treating head injuries as opposed to demonically caused physical maladies (Dimopoulos et al., 2008). More important for us and the study of health psychology is the connection that ancient physicians made between bodily humors and the psychology of individuals.

Humor theory is most often attributed to Hippocrates and later Galen, both ancient Greek physicians (Stelmack & Stalikas, 1991). The idea here is that when we think of medicine and the human body, we think of it as consisting of four main humors or bodily fluids. These bodily fluids are phlegm, black bile, yellow bile, and blood. Both Galen and Hippocrates, along with many other physicians, believed that these bodily fluids and their physical manifestations were very much tied to a person's temperament, or their personality characteristics. In Table 2.1, you can see how each humor represents certain physical components, as well as mental components, of a person's health. When you have too much humor, or not enough, you will become sick.

Table 2.1 Breakdown of Humors and Their Associated Characteristics

Humor	*Physical Manifestations*	*Psychological Characteristics*
Phlegm	Respiratory diseases Common cold Pneumonia	"Phlegmatic" Reserved Thoughtful Shy
Black bile	Dysentery Cholera Intestinal illness Cancer	"Melancholic" Sad Depressed Anxious Introspective
Yellow bile	Jaundice Inflammation of the skin	"Choleric" Driven Aggressive Impulsive
Blood	Anemia Fever	"Sanquine" Social Happy Full of energy

These fluids were seen to be intricately tied together with the physiological and the psychological. Even the words we use today to describe someone's psychological disposition come from humor theory: Someone who is "phlegmatic" is described as being calm and/or unemotional, someone who is "sanguine" is optimistic, a "melancholic" person is sad, whereas someone who is choleric is highly irritable.

Looking at Stephen King's characters through a humoral lens, you may be able to see how these dispositional types are represented. Let's take *The Shining,* for example, which we discussed in Chapter 1. Jack Torrence could easily be described as choleric – he is driven to finish his play, be the man of the house, but can also be over-aggressive, having physically harmed several people during bouts of anger. And this is even before the Overlook got hold of him. His body must be overrun with yellow bile!

The Dark Ages

Of course, humoral theory turned out to be not so accurate, but it was a good start in terms of physicians thinking about the mind–body connection. Unfortunately, these enlightened times did not last, and when we look at what was happening during the Middle Ages, we see that the "science" of the Ancient Greeks and Romans was replaced by mostly supernatural explanations of physical health and human psychology, dominated by the Church. This may fit right along with some Stephen King themes, but that is a discussion for another book.

Renaissance and Descartes

We did eventually move out of the Dark Ages, but in a sense, the real villain of health psychology was just entering the picture – René Descartes. René Descartes (1596–1650) was a French philosopher who famously stated, "I think, therefore I am." When Twitter first came on the scene, Stephen King humorously paraphrased Descartes (see Figure 2.3). Why Descartes is problematic for health

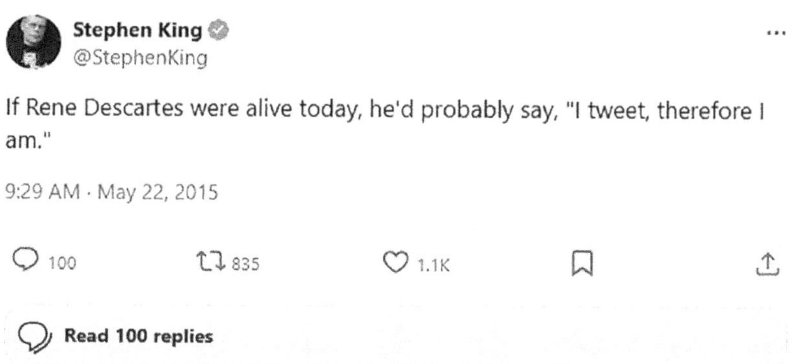
Stephen King
@StephenKing
If Rene Descartes were alive today, he'd probably say, "I tweet, therefore I am."
9:29 AM · May 22, 2015
100
835
1.1K
Read 100 replies

Figure 2.3 Stephen King Tweets About René Descartes Tweeting.

psychology is that he really codified the idea of Cartesian dualism, that the mind and body are independent, separate entities. While they can work together, they can also be completely independent of one another. This, of course, is a very watered-down interpretation of Descartes' philosophy, but you can see where it may have become popular with those who wished to study the body only. It makes things a lot easier when you are looking at health and disease to be able to say that only the body is important, and that is the only thing I need to look at. And indeed, that is what happened. Through these ideas, and the other innovations of the day, the biomedical model, which mostly discounts the mind, became the guiding principle of modern medicine.

Box 2.2 Miasma and *The Mist*

Prior to germ theory and the biomedical model, another disease theory consistently popped its head up – miasma theory. The idea here is that illnesses are caused by miasma – swaths of disease-riddled air to which people are exposed. This air could stem from "rotting" and "petrifying" (Kannadan, 2018) or any number of microscopic parasitic creepy-crawlies. These miasmas coming in and out of contact with humans created a wealth of societal ills – and were even theorized to be the source of a crime-riddled foggy 19th century London (Walters, 2019). In an absolutely fascinating article entitled "A Phantom on the Slum's Foul Air: Jack the Ripper and Miasma Theory," Walters described the connections that were made at the time between the infamous serial killer Jack the Ripper and the intense smell and heaviness of London's air and the miasmic theory of disease of the day. And indeed, I feel that any depiction of Jack the Ripper I have ever seen has shown a foggy, miasmic, dark London street, the air so thick you could cut it with a knife. The air, and the dangers within it, play a huge part in the story of Jack the Ripper and diseased-riddled London of the late 19th century. Of course, the areas of London exposed to these miasmatic forces were the poorest, and we will return to the topic of miasma in Chapter 6, when we discuss *The Running Man*.

The Jack the Ripper connection invokes the horror of Stephen King, but Stephen King himself has invoked the horror of miasma. Most of you Constant Readers out there know where I am going with this – King's novella – *The Mist* (King, 1985). In *The Mist*, a small town in Maine is engulfed by an extremely thick mist, which holds many hidden horrors. Of course, these horrors are not cholera or the simple plague, but they are definitely a hazard to your health – and life.

The Biomedical Model Begins

Once we left the Middle Ages, a new theme around health and medicine began to appear that still dominates to this day. Physicians and scientists began to focus on the purely biological and technical aspects of health and illness. Through this approach, humanity has made significant strides in how we prevent, treat, and cure illness. This period of time saw the invention of the microscope, X-rays, pasteurization, vaccines, penicillin, and on and on. Approaching health in this way is termed the Biomedical Model, and it still predominates in Western medicine.

This approach was much needed after the dark ages, and up until the first half of the last century, we had little understanding of the human body, and the techniques developed helped us to study the human body at levels never before possible. The ability to see viruses and bacteria under the lens of a microscope helped us to understand and conquer some of the most common killers of the past: influenza, tuberculosis, gastroenteritis, and so forth. These are what we would call acute disorders – they killed us fast and quickly, and in the US at least, the average lifespan in 1900 was 47 years. In 1918, when we experienced an influenza pandemic, the average age dropped to around 39 years. About 100 years later, in 2018, the average life span was almost 77 years (Kochanek et al., 2023). We have mostly the biomedical model to thank for those almost 40 extra years.

Breuer, Freud, Alexandar, and Dunbar – Psychosomatic Medicine Fights Back

While everyone was busy pasteurizing milk, building X-ray machines, and injecting small boys with cowpox to create vaccines,[2] two physicians in Vienna were wondering why they couldn't figure out what was wrong with a certain subset of their patients. One of these physicians was Joseph Breuer, and he was particularly concerned about his patient, Anna O.[3] At one point in her life, Anna O developed crippling physical symptoms, such as paralysis, and had trouble speaking. However, a "biomedical" explanation for why this was occurring could not be found.

Instead of using the common biological-focused treatment of the day, Breuer began using the "talking cure" – when she could talk, he let her discuss fictional stories to allow her to process her distress (Launer, 2005). Since her symptoms began after her father had died, much of the "talking" revolved around her trauma. According to the work published by Breuer and his then mentee Sigmund Freud, this work was able to resolve her physical symptoms (and she was able to become an extremely important figure in history in her own right – see Box 2.3). The argument was then that in order to treat some patients with physical symptoms, the mind had to be taken into account.

Box 2.3 Anna O Is Bertha Pappenheim, and Rose Madder?

In the 1950s, a Freud biographer revealed that Anna O was a woman named Bertha Pappenheim, who had died in 1936.[4] As a social worker, I am indebted to the foundational work that Pappenheim did for that field (Jusko, 2025). She became a feminist and social reformer who founded the German Jewish Women's Association. She also believed that women had the power to fix the social problems of the day and worked tirelessly to empower the women around her.

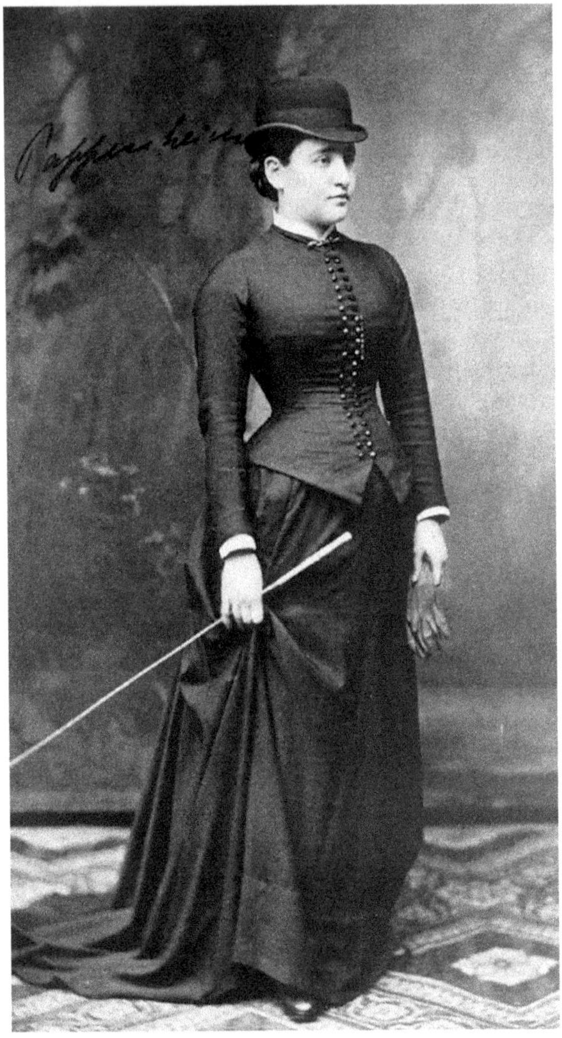

Figure 2.4 Image of Bertha Pappenheim, aka Anna O.

Bertha Pappenheim, and her transformation from Anna O to an empowered feminist, reminds me of several female Stephen King characters that overcame traumas of their male-dominated societies to become their own person, and reach potentials they were kept from achieving. The one that I can't help thinking about here is Rose Daniels, the protagonist of King's 1995 novel *Rose Madder*. She goes from timid and abused Rosie Daniels, wife of Norman, to independent and successful Rose McClendon, to the powerful Rosie Real. All while working with the women of the Daughters and Sisters shelter and finding her path to herself.

When I think of these strong women, who overcome so much adversity, that inhabit the world of Stephen King (e.g., Beverly Marsh, Delores Claiborne, Susannah Dean), I can't help but think of King's description of his own mother. According to King's own account, Nellie Ruth Pillsbury King was an amazing and supportive mother, giving him the confidence to be who he could be, despite their life circumstances. She provided all this support even in the face of being abandoned by her husband, raising two kids on her own, and working numerous low-paying and back-breaking jobs. Until she died of cancer at the age of 59, she was the epitome of the strong woman who overcomes what life throws at her, and this seems to permeate much of Stephen King's writing.

From this work with Anna O and many others, Freud went on to formulate an explanation which he called conversion disorder – the idea that when a patient is experiencing physical symptoms with no known biological or organic basis, they may be physically manifesting unconscious conflict (Ali et al., 2015). In essence, matters of the mind are manifesting themselves in the body.

Unfortunately for Breuer, the student eclipsed the teacher in popularity, and the work of Freud caught fire, and he is who we mainly think about when we think about the "talking cure." There were, of course, a lot of critics, especially those wed to the biomedical model. Yet others in the medical community saw the potential in starting to incorporate the mind more in treating medical conditions, especially as infectious diseases became less of a concern.

Enter Helen Flanders Dunbar and Franz Alexander – the honorary mother and father of psychosomatic medicine. The word "psychosomatic" comes from two Greek words – psyche, of course, meaning "mind" and soma meaning "body." Psychosomatic medicine became the branch of medicine that fought back against the biomedical model, especially given the work of Breuer, Freud, and others. In 1932, Dunbar founded a new medical journal, called "Psychosomatic Medicine," which then led to the founding of the American Society for Research in Psychosomatic Problems in 1942, which eventually became the American Psychosomatic Society, or simply, APS (Herrmann-Lingen, 2017).[5] APS is important to note, because as Lovallo points out, it "was one of the first medical societies to be dedicated to the integration of biology, psychology, and social factors" (Lovallo, 2010). A small subsection of medical professionals was starting to see that there may be more to practicing medicine than what is incorporated into the biomedical model.

While working alongside Dunbar in the founding of the journal and the society, Alexander wrote the book "Psychosomatic Medicine: Its Principles and Applications," in 1950, which became the guiding textbook of psychosomatic medicine practitioners. In it, he describes what he considered the "Holy Seven Psychosomatic Diseases" (see Box 2.4) – diseases in which biological or organic explanations currently elude doctors practicing the biomedical model and thus justify a more exact mind–body science.

Box 2.4 The Holy Seven Psychosomatic Diseases

Peptic Ulcer
Bronchial Asthma
Rheumatoid Arthritis
Ulcerative Colitis
Essential Hypertension
Neurodermatitis
Thyrotoxicosis

The work of Dunbar and Alexander helped the mind–body movement make huge inroads into the dominant biomedical model. Yet there are a few more big names – Walter Cannon and Hans Selye – that helped the medical establishment to see even further outside of the box, and to get us even closer to the founding of health psychology in the 1970s.

Thinking Outside of the Biomedical Model – Walter Cannon

Just a few decades before King's birth, some important foundational work was being done in terms of how we think about psychology affecting the body, and the HPA axis that we talked about in Chapter 1. One of the most important figures at this time was Walter Cannon, a Harvard-trained physician who was instrumental in understanding how emotions are associated with psychological arousal. He studied this fight or flight response in a way that allows me to explain exactly what happened to me while reading *The Shining*. We will discuss these scientific techniques used by Cannon and others in Chapter 3 when we tackle the research methods of health psychology.

Interestingly enough, Walter Cannon may have gone the way of the biomedical model, as early in his medical career, he utilized those body-focused innovative X-rays to study digestion. Yet Cannon was too much of an adventurer for that – later in Chapter 4, you will see his forays into other cultures and beliefs, with his research on voodoo curses. Later on in his career, he switched from being interested in digestion to being interested in emotions and fight or flight mechanisms. From his laboratory at Harvard Medical School, he produced research looking at how the emotions of fear or threat could instigate adrenal pathways (what we now refer to as the SAM axis; see Chapter 1) (Cannon & De La Paz, 1911).

From here, he began to make connections from emotions to disease and became more concerned with the clinical implications of his work (Brown & Fee, 2002). The fact that he worked as a physiologist, using the latest in biological measurement technology, certainly lent an air of legitimacy to the psychosomatic medicine movement. We can also thank Walter Cannon for helping us better understand why we love to be scared, and why many of us gravitate toward Stephen King.

Health, Stress, and the Birth of Stephen King

A year after Stephen King was born, the World Health Organization (WHO) published its definition of "health." This is a significant turning point for this book in many ways. One, of course, is that it is happening right around the time of King's birth. The second important point is that this newly adopted definition of health goes far beyond what would be encompassed in the biomedical model. This definition, which is still in use today, states that:

> Health is a state of complete physical, mental, and social well-being, and not merely the absences of disease or infirmity.
>
> (WHO, 1948)

This means that health is far more than not being sick, and the implications of this are vast. Now we get to the point in time where Stephen King and health psychology begin to overlap.

A few years after that, another huge figure came on the scene – Hans Selye. While Walter Cannon may have been the first to publicly use the word stress, it was Selye who is known as the father of stress research, and the one who really brought it to the public's attention right around the time Stephen King was growing up. For how pervasive the word is in our current day and age, you may be shocked to find out that it did not enter our common parlance until the 1950s. When King was around eight or nine years old, Hans Selye published his book *The Stress of Life* (Selye, 1956) and published an article in Science (Selye, 1955) that would lay out his ideas linking stress and health.

One can't help but think that the popularization of the concept of stress in the 1950s played a role in the work of Stephen King. Bev Vincent, one of King's biographers, has stated that "… one of the secrets of King's success – (is that) his books are fundamentally about how people react to stressful circumstances" (Vincent, 2022, p.37). Our, and King's, understanding of what stressful circumstances are, and how they can impact our bodies, is largely due to Selye.

One of the biggest contributions of Selye's work was the idea that severe and/or prolonged stress exposure can wear down the body. First, Selye defined stress as any demand placed upon the body that causes the body to respond. In his vision of stress, any demand placed upon the mind or body would create a non-specific body response (Tan & Yip, 2018). The body would then have to work on creating a balance within itself, while the demand was still present. Hopefully, the demand, or stressor, would resolve itself quickly – but if it did not and the body had to keep accounting for it, then the body systems would eventually become exhausted. It is within the exhaustive state, resulting from stress, that we then become vulnerable to disease, illness, poor health habits, and so forth.

We will talk more about Selye when we discuss psychoneuroimmunology in *The Stand* in Chapter 8, but it is important to note that the work of Cannon and Selye, along with the WHO's new definition of health, set the stage for health psychology to come into being in the 1970s, along with the now-famous writer, Stephen King.

The 1970s – Stephen King, the Biopsychosocial Model, and Health Psychology Make Themselves Known

We will start our journey into the 1970s by talking about King, since we seem to have left him a bit behind in the last few sections (it didn't help that he hadn't been born yet, but that is neither here nor there). While the WHO was determining what we mean by health, and Selye was figuring out the mechanisms of stress, King was starting to explore his writing chops. In the late 1950s, his brother Dave started a newspaper (mostly for the neighbors) called "Dave's Rag," of which King was a standard (though young) contributor. As he got a bit older (if you can consider 13 older), he began to submit his short stories to various magazines and consequently received various rejections. In high school, he did get a few stories published in the school newspaper, and he got his "big break" in 1963, when a magazine called *Comics Review* published his short story "I Was a Teenage Grave Robber." He was only 16, so in my book, this wasn't too shabby.

He graduated from high school in 1966 and attended the University of Maine at Orono until he graduated in 1970. A lot of stuff happened during this time, don't get me wrong – he met and married his wife, he struggled with writing and working, and making money to support his family. But you can read all about that in the books dedicated to exploring his life, like Bev Vincent's *Stephen King: A Complete Exploration of His Work, Life, and Influences* (2022).

What we care about is when the world started to know Stephen King – and that came with the 1974 publication of the novel *Carrie*. This initial printing and the $2,500 paycheck weren't earth-shattering, but when the paperback rights were sold for a quarter of a million dollars, we could safely say that Stephen King had ARRIVED. The money made it so that King could write full-time, and *Salem's Lot*, *The Shining*, and *The Stand* all arrived by 1978.

Now back to health psychology – for while King was making a name for himself, so was the biopsychosocial model. While this was not the first time a biopsychosocial approach had been broached, it was George Engel's 1977 *Science* article "The Need for a New Medical Model: A Challenge for Biomedicine" that truly brought it to the forefront. The idea that someone published, in *Science* no less, a paper outlining the significant shortcomings of the biomedical model, was ground-breaking (much like the book *Carrie* was to many horror fans). The 1970s certainly were mixing things up!

Along with this new embrace of the biopsychosocial model, some people within the field started to shy away from certain aspects of psychosomatic medicine, particularly the aspects that were beholden to the strong Freudian ideas of the unconscious causes of illness and disease, and the limiting ideas of psychosomatic medicine only applying to the Holy Seven. Researchers and clinicians began to think that it was a much more complex phenomenon, and that neither the unconscious components of psychoanalysis nor the purely biomedical model was sufficient. They were looking for a new field that would truly incorporate all of the

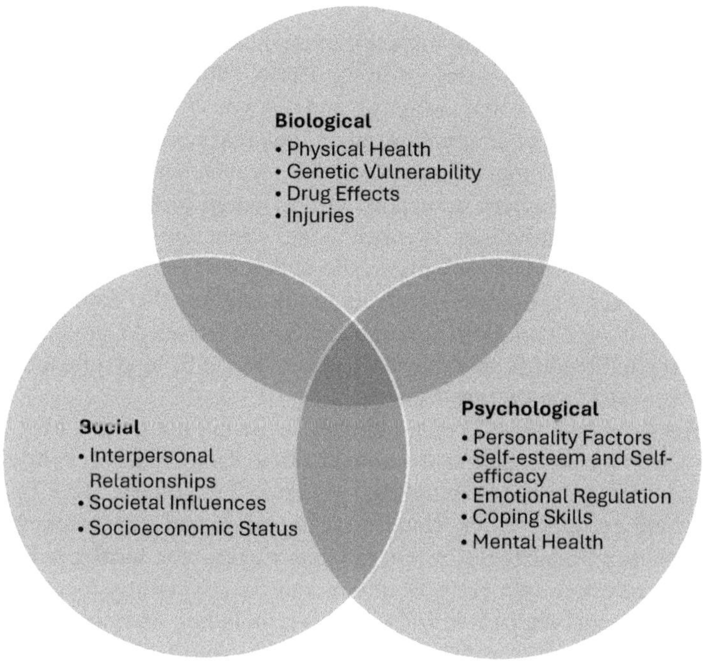

Figure 2.5 Graphic Representation of Factors Included in the Biopsychosocial Model.

aspects of the biopsychosocial model (see Figure 2.5 for an illustration of the factors that the biopsychosocial model could entail).

Those who wished to move away from the purely psychosomatic model moved toward what this book is all about – health psychology (phew, we finally got there!). Just to show you how new a field health psychology is, the American Psychological Association (APA) was founded in 1892. As subfields were developed, the APA formed subdivisions – for example, Division 1 is the Society for General Psychology and Interdisciplinary Inquiry, Division 2 is the Society for the Teaching of Psychology. Division 38 – the Society for Health Psychology – was officially recognized in 1978. Again, the 1970s for the win!

Box 2.5 Collaborations: King, Health Psychology, and the Pittsburgh Connection

There is a huge part in the history of health psychology that we are missing here – the fact that scientists, since the formation of Division 38, have spent decades formulating the theories, collecting the data, and disseminating the findings that now make up the backbone of our field. Of course, I will be presenting a large amount of this work throughout this book, but if we want to think about what was going on in the 1980s, 1990s, and beyond, we can think about important collaborations – and that goes for Stephen King, too!

The collaborations I am thinking about took place in Pittsburgh, Pennsylvania, my adoptive home. Let's start off with Stephen King. In 1981, Stephen King and George Romero descended on Pittsburgh to film *Creepshow* – a five-story horror anthology. Stephen King wrote the story, and George Romero was the director. Joining in the collab was Pittsburgh native Tom Savini, the make-up and special effects genius behind other Romero classics like *Dawn of the Dead*. Both Romero and Savini attended Carnegie Mellon University in Pittsburgh, and they drafted another CMU alum into the Creepshow mix – Ted Danson (pre-Cheers).

While King was the odd man out here, as he did not go to CMU or live in Pittsburgh for any significant amount of time, he did take on a little bit of the lingo, what we call Pittsburghese. In Figure 2.6, you can see a Tweet by King where he refers to his Romero collaboration and uses some Grade A Pittsburghese ("Jaunt Iggle" refers to Giant Eagle – the local grocery store chain). Needless to say, King, Romero, and Savini coming together made some great things happen with *Creepshow*, including Stephen King really chewing up the scenery as the character of Jordy Verrill. This Pittsburgh collaboration was exciting to most horror fans, with Cinefantastique Magazine putting King, Romero, and Savini on the front cover of their September/October 1982 issue with the caption "Are These the Scariest Men in America?" (Gagne, 1982).

On the health psychology side, we have another amazing Pittsburgh collaboration in the Pittsburgh Mind–Body Center (PMBC) – where researchers from the University of Pittsburgh and Carnegie Mellon University came together to plan, fund, conduct, and publish some major milestones in health psychology. This also included a training program (Cardiovascular Behavioral Medicine Program) that has produced some of the biggest names in health psychology research.

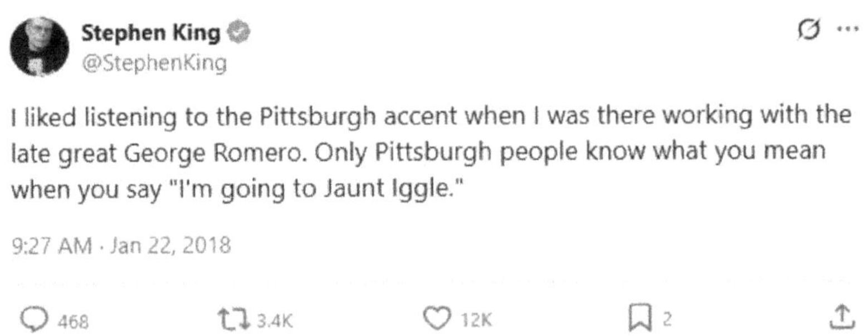
Stephen King
@StephenKing
I liked listening to the Pittsburgh accent when I was there working with the late great George Romero. Only Pittsburgh people know what you mean when you say "I'm going to Jaunt Iggle."
9:27 AM · Jan 22, 2018
468
3.4K
12K
2

Figure 2.6 Stephen king Tweets About George Romero and Pittsburgh.

This collab happened about a decade after *Creepshow*, with Dr. Karen Matthews at Pitt and Dr. Michael Scheier at CMU cofounding the center. Much of the research we will discuss in this book, particularly the common cold findings in *The Stand* chapter, as well as much of the cardiovascular work, was made possible by the PMBC. While most of the top researchers and scientists involved in these collaborations have since retired, other researchers in Pittsburgh have taken up the mantle, creating the Health Psych Research Network, which continues to produce world-class research and keep the PMBC legacy going strong (much like *Creepshow 2*).

Just like Stephen King's career, health psychology took off as a discipline. Hence, my ability to write a book about both! Health psychology today is a thriving field, and its goals, especially given what we have experienced over the past several years with COVID-19, have never been more important. What are those goals? In one of the most widely used health psychology textbooks in the world (Taylor & Stanton, 2021), the goals are listed as follows:

1 To focus on promoting healthy lifestyles and maintaining those lifestyles
2 To prevent and treat illness
3 To understand the etiology (origins or causes) and association of health, disease, and dysfunction.
4 Understand and improve how health care is provided and received.

Luckily for us, all of this and more are demonstrated throughout the works of Stephen King. Was he influenced by all that was taking place in the battle between the biomedical model, psychosomatic medicine, and the biopsychosocial model that occurred in his lifetime? We would have to ask him that (hey Steve, call me anytime!), but I think that so much of what we discuss in health psychology is just an essential part of human struggle and triumph, and Stephen King is just attuned to those things in general. It makes sense to me that these two would go hand in hand.

Health Psychology, Writing, and Stephen King

Before we move on to specific works of King and health psychology topics, I want to provide one more example of the connection between the two.

We can't ignore one area of huge overlap between Stephen King and health psychology: expressive writing. While expressive writing was first proposed in a health psychology context by James Pennebaker in the 1980s, the ideas underlying the "writing cure" were very much part of Breuer and Freud's "talking cure" that we discussed earlier (Lepore & Smyth, 2002). The idea here is that in order to process – or work through – traumatic, emotional experiences, you must express them – either by talking them out or by writing them down.

Expressive writing is a form of writing in which people are asked to think about the most stressful or traumatic experiences of their lives (Pennebaker, 1997). They are then told to write, for approximately 20 minutes, about the event and the feelings and thoughts they have about it. They are told not to worry about making spelling or grammar mistakes, and they are asked to repeat the task over several sessions. In my personal opinion, one of the hardest parts of the tasks is that you can't stop – you have to keep going for the full 20 minutes. Yet you can rest assured that by the time you are done, you have gotten all the emotions out.

To test the efficacy of these expressive writing interventions, randomized controlled trials are conducted. I will discuss exactly what happens in these clinical trials in more detail in Chapter 3, but know that the research on expressive writing and health has been quite striking. An early meta-analysis (Smyth, 1998) showed that in the long term, those who were randomized to the expressive writing group showed significant improvement in reported health, psychological well-being, physiological functioning, and overall functioning. It is important to note that when actually doing the writing tasks, those writing about traumatic events had a significant increase in distress levels compared to those writing about things like breakfast. This is to be expected, as they are bringing up painful and distressing feelings – but over time, doing so helped to improve their health in significant ways.

Expressive writing becomes an important concept in our Stephen King discussion due to what occurred on June 19th, 1999. On that day, Stephen King was handed a traumatic experience worthy of the expressive writing task – he was hit by a minivan while walking and came very close to losing his life. His leg was broken in almost a dozen places, his lung collapsed on the way to the hospital, he also broke his hip and four ribs, several places in his spine were "chipped," and his head required 30 stitches (King, June 2000).

The accident itself was traumatic, but so was the road to recovery after. Yet, five weeks after the accident, King was back to writing. He stated, "I had been in terrible situations before, and writing had helped me get over them" (King, June 2000). He also states that writing "can be a way back to life." I think his sentiments connect deeply to what Freud and Breuer referred to in the talking cure, and what Pennebaker and others were getting at with the idea of the writing cure.

Some of you may argue that by getting back to his novels and short stories, he was not actually participating in expressive writing – as he was not writing about his own trauma. However, we can see points where he is – The *New Yorker* article I just quoted, for one (this was also included as the postscript in his book *On Writing: A Memoir of the Craft*). Those are fairly obvious examples of King writing about his traumas. For those of you who are "ka-tet," you know that he also writes about this event in book seven of *The Dark Tower* series. Here, King makes the accident an important part of Roland of Gilead's quest. I hope that just like the participants in the expressive writing studies, he found increased physical health and mental well-being from having written so much about that day in 1999. I think the act of writing, and what it can do for your health and well-being (as well as reading!), is a key part of what this book is about.

Where We Are Today

Health psychology, and thank goodness Stephen King, are still going strong today. Psychosomatic medicine and health psychology are trying to find their way back to one another. For example, in 2024, the American Psychosomatic Society was renamed the Society for Biopsychosocial Science and Medicine. The fields involved in the formation of health psychology are becoming more proactive in terms of health policies and health care improvement, focusing not just on research, but also on applied proactive health innovations. And Stephen King himself has not faded from public view – within the last few months of writing this book, he has published a new novel called *Never Flinch* and had his short story "Life of Chuck" and his book *The Long Walk* adapted into films that were recently released, and next month, both the TV show *Welcome to Derry* (based on *It*) and a new movie adaptation of *The Running Man* will be released. It is an exciting time to be both a fan of health psychology and Stephen King, which I hope this book will convince you to be!

Stephen King Memoirs and Biographies

Memoir Book: King, S. (2000). *Stephen King on Writing: A Memoir on the Craft to On Writing: A Memoir of the Craft*. Scribner.

Memoir Audiobook: King, S. (2000). *On Writing: A Memoir of the Craft* [Audiobook]. Simon & Schuster Audio. https://www.audible.com/pd/On-Writing-Audiobook/B002V0A5DK

Biography: Rogak, L. (2009). *Haunted Heart: The Life and Times of Stephen King*. Thomas Dunne Books.

Biography: Vincent, B. (2022). *Stephen King: A Complete Exploration of His Work, life, and influences.* Epic Ink.

Learn More Questions

1 The manifestations of the humoral theory can be seen throughout the character development in most of Stephen King's novels and short stories. Can you find some good examples? Using the table presented in Table 2.1 as a template, create a humoral table of Stephen King characters. Does it align well with what Hippocrates and Galen theorized?
2 Beyond *The Dark Tower*, identify and analyze other works by Stephen King, in which he appears to be processing personal or emotional life experiences through storytelling. How do these experiences shape the themes, characters, or narrative structure of the work(s)? Consider how King uses horror, fantasy, or psychological elements to explore grief, addiction, fear, or recovery. Support your analysis with specific examples from the text(s).
3 What other instances of miasma-type horrors can you see in the work of Stephen King? How do they tie in with how the miasma theory attempted to understand public health?

Notes

1 You will see two dips in the data where life expectancy lowered a bit – one was during the Spanish Flu Epidemic of 1918, and the other (starting in 2020) was COVID-19-related.
2 Yes, this really happened – in the late 18th century, a scientist named Edward Jenner was trying to figure out how to fight smallpox, which was killing a lot of people at the time. He thought that maybe he could take the pus from a milder form of pox – cowpox – and inject it into someone, and it could help them fight off smallpox. So he did just that, injecting the eight-year-old son of his gardener with the pus from the wounds of a milk-maid with cowpox. As far as we know, it worked, and the boy did not get smallpox. Thus, we have the first vaccine – with the word itself stemming from the Latin for cow (female) – vacca (Turley, 2021).
3 Anna O is a pseudonym that was used when Breuer and Freud opted to publish their experiences treating Anna. Pseudonyms are used to protect the patient's confidentiality, and Anna O isn't the only famous pseudonym in psychology. For example, in cognitive psychology, we have HM, a patient who had parts of his hippocampus removed to prevent seizures. He was unable to form new (declarative) memories after the procedure, which helped scientists understand that multiple types of memory exist.
4 In most cases, after a patient with a pseudonym dies, their real identity is revealed, as long as the family agrees. For example, after his death in 2008, HM was revealed to be Henry Molaison. I like knowing their names, as we have much to thank these pioneering patients for, and their names deserve our respect.
5 Full disclosure – I have been a member of APS since I started my PhD in 2008. However, acknowledging some of the ways our field has moved beyond the psychosomatic, as it is described here, the society voted to change its name in 2024, and is now the Society for Biopsychosocial Science and Medicine, or SBSM (Gianaros et al., 2025).

Bibliography

Ahmad, F. B., Cisewski, J. A., & Anderson, R. N. (2024). Leading causes of death in the US, 2019–2023. *JAMA, 332*(12), 957–958. https://doi.org/10.1001/jama.2024.15563

Alexander, F. (1950). *Psychosomatic medicine: Its principles and applications.* W. W. Norton & Co.

Ali, S., Jabeen, S., Pate, R. J., Shahid, M., Chinala, S., Nathani, M., & Shah, R. (2015). Conversion disorder—mind versus body: A review. *Innovations in Clinical Neuroscience, 12*(5–6), 27–33. PMID: 26155375.

Brown, T. M., & Fee, E. (2002). Walter Bradford Cannon: Pioneer physiologist of human emotions. *American Journal of Public Health, 92*(10), 1594–1595. https://doi.org/10.2105/AJPH.92.10.1594

Cannon, W. B. & de la Paz, D. (1911). Emotional stimulation of adrenal secretion. *American Journal of Physiology, 28* (1), 64–70. https://doi.org/10.1152/ajplegacy.1911.28.1.64

Dimopoulos, V. G., Robinson III, J. S., & Fountas, K. N. (2008). The pearls and pitfalls of skull trephination as described in the hippocratic treatise "On Head Wounds". *Journal of the History of the Neurosciences, 17*(2), 131–140. https://doi.org/10.1080/09647040701296770

Engel, G. L. (1977). The need for a new medical model: A challenge for biomedicine. *Science (American Association for the Advancement of Science), 196*(4286), 129–136. https://doi.org/10.1126/science.847460

Fabbri, P. F., Lonoce, N., Masieri, M., Caramella, D., Valentino, M., & Vassallo, S. (2012). Partial cranial trephination by means of Hippocrates' trypanon from 5th century BC Himera (Sicily, Italy). *International Journal of Osteoarchaeology, 22*(2), 194–200. https://doi.org/10.1002/oa.1197

Gagne, P. R. (1982, September/October). Creepshow: It's an $8 million comic book, from George Romero & friends. *Cinefantastique*, *13*(1), 17–35.

Gianaros, P. J., Lewis, T. T., Segerstrom, S. C., Tomiyama, A. J., & Gruenewald, T. L. (2025). Towards a second social movement in biopsychosocial science and medicine. *Biopsychosocial Science and Medicine, 87*(1), 2–3. https://doi.org/10.1097/PSY.0000000000001362

Helmore, E. (2000, October). The writer, the accident, and the lonely end. *The Guardian.*

Herrmann-Lingen, C. (2017). The American psychosomatic society–integrating mind, brain, body and social context in medicine since 1942. *BioPsychoSocial Medicine, 11*, 1–7. https://doi.org/10.1186/s13030-017-0096-6

Johnson, B. T., & Acabchuk, R. L. (2018). What are the keys to a longer, happier life? Answers from five decades of health psychology research. *Social Science & Medicine* (1982), *196*, 218–226. https://doi.org/10.1016/j.socscimed.2017.11.001

Jusko, P. (2025). Between therapy, activism, and profession: Bertha Pappenheim's contribution to the formation of modern social work. *IOSR Journal of Humanities and Social Sciences, 30*(7,5), 6 13.

Kannadan, A. (2018). History of the miasma theory of disease. *Essai, 16*(1), 18. https://dc.cod.edu/essai/vol16/iss1/18

King, S. (1985). *The Mist.* In *Skeleton Crew*. Putnam.

King, S. (2000). *Stephen King on Writing: A Memoir on the Craft to On Writing: A Memoir of the Craft.* Scribner.

King, S. (2000, June 11). *On impact: After an accidents, learning to write again. The New Yorker.*

Kochanek, K. D., Murphy, S. L., Xu, J., & Arias, E. (2023). Deaths: Final Data for 2020. National vital statistics reports : From the Centers for Disease Control and Prevention, National Center for Health Statistics, National Vital Statistics System, 72(10), 1–92. PMID: 37748091.

Launer, J. (2005). Anna O and the 'talking cure'. *QJM, 98*(6), 465–466. https://doi.org/10.1093/qjmed/hci068

Lepore, S. J., & Smyth, J. M. (Eds.). (2002). *The writing cure: How expressive writing promotes health and emotional well-being.* American Psychological Association. https://doi.org/10.1037/10451-000

Levenson, D. (1994). *Mind, body, and medicine: A history of the American Psychosomatic Society.* American Psychosomatic Society.

Lovallo, W. R. (2010). American Psychosomatic Society. *The Corsini Encyclopedia of Psychology, 1*(1), 84. https://doi.org/10.1002/9780470479216.corpsy0722

Maier, K. J. (2025). Becoming biopsychosocial toward comprehensive health for 21st century science and medicine. *Biopsychosocial Science and Medicine, 87*(1), 4–6. https://doi.org/10.1097/psy.0000000000001361

McKeown, R. E. (2009). The epidemiologic transition: Changing patterns of mortality and population dynamics. *American Journal of Lifestyle Medicine*, *3*(1 Suppl), 19S–26S. https://doi.org/10.1177/1559827609335350

Murray, M. (2014). Social history of health psychology: Context and textbooks. *Health Psychology Review, 8*(2), 215–237. https://doi.org/10.1080/17437199.2012.701058

Nanayakkara, S., & Gunarathne, M. S. (2022). New insights on the surgical procedure of trephination throughout human history. *Archaeology*, *2*(1), 1–9. https://doi.org/10.47509/JHAA.2022.v02i01.01

Pennebaker, J. W. (1997). Writing about emotional experiences as a therapeutic process. *Psychological Science*, *8*(3), 162–166. https://doi.org/10.1111/j.1467-9280.1997.tb00403.x

Selye, H. (1955). Stress and disease. *Science, 122*(3171), 625–631. https://doi.org/10.1126/science.122.3171.625

Selye, H. (1956). *The stress of life*. New York: McGraw-hill.Smyth, J. M. (1998). Written emotional expression: Effect sizes, outcome types, and moderating variables. *Journal of Consulting and Clinical Psychology*, *66*(1), 174. https://doi.org/10.1037/0022-006X.66.1.174

Smyth, J., & Helm, R. (2003). Focused expressive writing as self-help for stress and trauma. *Journal of Clinical Psychology*, *59*(2), 227–235. https://doi.org/10.1002/jclp.10144

Stelmack, R. M., & Stalikas, A. (1991). Galen and the humour theory of temperament. *Personality and Individual Differences, 12*(3), 255–263. https://doi.org/10.1016/0191-8869(91)90111-N

Tan, S. Y., & Yip, A. (2018). Hans Selye (1907–1982): Founder of the stress theory. *Singapore Medical Journal*, *59*(4), 170. https://doi.org/10.11622/smedj.2018043

Taylor, S. E., & Stanton, A. L. (2021). *Health psychology*. McGraw-Hill Higher Education.

Turley P. K. (2021). Vaccine: From *vacca,* a cow. *AJO-DO Clinical Companion, 1*(1), 5–6. https://doi.org/10.1016/j.xaor.2021.02.005

Vincent, B. (2022). *Stephen King: A complete exploration of his work, life, and influences.* Epic Ink.

Walters, D. W. (2019). A Phantom on the Slum's Foul Air: Jack the Ripper and Miasma Theory. *Victorian Periodicals Review*, *52*(3), 588–603. https://doi.org/10.1353/vpr.2019.0036

World Health Organization (1948). Summary Reports on Proceedings Minutes and Final Acts of the International Health Conference held in New York from 19 June to 22 July 1946. *World Health Organization*, available from: https://apps.who.int/iris/handle/10665/85573

3 Measuring Your Fear

Research Methods in Health Psychology

Health Psychology Is Evidence-Based

Health psychology is a scientific endeavor – that is we use research to gather evidence in order to form our hypotheses, theories, and ultimately our recommendations for clinical interventions. In a sense, we are grounded in realism – that is what is actually occurring in the real world. This may seem the exact antithesis of what Stephen King is all about, and I think that may be true – which makes this research methods chapter particularly difficult!

I am going to put my best foot forward here to teach you about some of the research methods used in health psychology, but with a Stephen King slant. The most obvious example that comes to my mind when I think of an evidence-based character in Stephen King's work is Louis Creed from *Pet Sematary* (see Box 3.1 for summary).

Box 3.1 ***Pet Sematary***

Stephen King's *Pet Sematary* was published in 1983, after spending a few years hidden away (see Box 3.2). Yet ever since its publication, it has been teaching many of us that "sometimes, dead is better," through the best-selling book itself, two film adaptations (1989 and 2019), a sequel (*Pet Sematary* Two, 1992), and a prequel (*Pet Sematary: Bloodlines*, 2023).

The novel follows Louis Creed, a doctor who moves his family (wife Rachel, daughter Ellie, and son Gage) from Chicago to Maine so that he can take over as medical director of university health services at the University of Maine. As much as Rachel and Louis love their new house, it is located on a very busy road that is a potential raceway for speeding cars and trucks. While this presents a very real danger to their pets (particularly their roaming tomboy cat Winston Churchill, or Church for short) and children, there are other more mythical places of danger surrounding them.

After becoming very close with their older neighbors across the street – Jud and Norma Crandell – Jud takes the Creeds on a hiking trip to

DOI: 10.4324/9781003495994-3

the "Pet Sematary," which is located somewhat deep in the woods by their home. This is where the children of the town have been taking their dead pets for burial for generations, and a misspelled sign marks the spot of the rituals.

⚠ **[Spoiler Alert]** Shortly after the trip to the Pet Sematary, the University starts its fall semester. On the very first day of classes, Louis experiences the death of a student at the medical center, when Victor Pascow is brought in after being hit by a car while riding his bike. Right before Victor dies in front of Louis, he tells him that the Pet Sematary is not the real cemetery, and to "keep clear." The next night, Victor visits him and tells him, "The door must not be opened."

While initially disturbed by the Pascow incident, Louis is able to rationalize it away, and things eventually calm down, and his work at the center becomes less dramatic and more mundane. The fall goes by, and the Creeds continue their close relationship with the Crandells – with Louis coming to see Jud as the father he never had. During the excitement of Halloween, Norma has a heart attack – and the quick thinking of Louis prevents it from being fatal. It is because of this that Jud attempts a very misguided thank you that starts the true horror of the book.

As foreshadowed when the Creeds first move to busy highway U.S. Route 1 – Church, the cat, is found dead after getting hit by a car. This occurs when Rachel, Ellie, and Gage are at Louis's in-laws for Thanksgiving, and he has stayed behind to work. Louis is devastated that he will have to tell Ellie that her beloved cat is dead. Sensing his devastation and wanting to pay him back for saving his wife's life – Jud takes Louis and the body of Church to the burial ground beyond the Pet Sematary. Located a few harrowing miles beyond is an ancient burial ground – where if you bury something, it will become reanimated. Jud once took his dog there, and now he shows Louis what to do, to spare Ellie the pain of losing her cat.

And indeed, who comes waltzing in the next afternoon – Church. He comes back a bit different, a bit smelly, but he is back just the same. While Jud has prevented Louis from having to deliver the difficult news of the death of the family pet, he has set into motion something far more devastating. His mistake becomes clear to him when Gage, who has just learned to walk, gets hit by a speeding truck and suffers the same fate as Church.

Blinded by grief over the loss of his son, Louis does the unthinkable and takes Gage's body to the burial ground beyond the Pet Sematary. Despite being told of a time when a young man named Timmy Baterman was buried there, and how he did not come back as he once was – Louis is more hopeful. He shouldn't have been – the Gage that returns is evil, and murders Jud and Rachel, and Louis is forced to kill the son he hoped would return to him. There is more, but I will leave it to you to find out what happens next!

Louis Creed – Man of Science

When we first meet Louis Creed at the beginning of *Pet Sematary*, he is highly dedicated to empiricism and the scientific method. His world is grounded in the reality of facts, the weight of evidence, and finding the rational, plausible, and most empirical explanations for the occurrences of life. As a medical doctor, we assume that Louis abides by the scientific method – a process by which the world is observed, questions are asked, predictions are made, data are collected, conclusions are made, and then the process repeats with the new information. Within this process, we develop theories and hypotheses – theories are the larger explanations we gather from phenomena, while the hypotheses are the more specific statement/question/prediction that stem from theories and/or help them become more refined. For example, in this book, we will look at hypotheses that stem from theories such as the theory of planned behavior (Ajzen, 1991), social cognitive theory (Bandura, 2013), and the minority stress theory (Meyer, 2003).

I would argue that at the beginning of *Pet Sematary*, Louis Creed has a pretty strong theory that "dead is dead" – once you have died, you will remain in that state indefinitely (it's science!). He also believes that when it comes to being dead or not dead, being "not dead" is preferable, and as a medical doctor, his goal is to make sure that everyone stays alive. However, Jud Crandall puts forth a hypothesis that might upset Louis' theory. The hypothesis of course being "… sometimes dead is better" (King, 2014, p.208). Louis then spends the rest of the novel gathering evidence against Jud's statement, to keep his theory intact. I will leave it to the reader to interpret the results.

Where the Evidence Comes From

In several scenes within the book, we see Louis immersing himself in medical literature, or discussing possible case studies he can present at conferences, and so forth. In an attempt to thwart sleep, he is seen "reading a stack of medical journals" (King, 2014, p.118). After the incident with Victor Pascow, he travels to a conference and presents a paper on the legalities of treating students. Conferences and journal articles are all key parts of the scientific endeavor – it is through these that researchers get their findings out there (except when those findings are null; see Box 3.2). When it comes to conducting research, what is found, or not found, needs to be shared in order for us to make progress in our understanding. Preliminarily, you might take your findings to a conference, to share among your peers. Once you receive feedback and interest at a conference, then it might be time to send it out to a wider audience, via a peer-reviewed journal.

What do we mean by peer review? It generally looks like this – after researchers have conducted a study and analyzed the data, they will write up the results in a standard journal article format (see Table 3.1). They will choose what journal to send it to, and then it will go to that journal's editor. The editor will then make an initial decision on whether the paper is a good fit for the journal. If they decide yes, then they will send it off to three other researchers who are considered experts in the type of research/topic being discussed. These "peer reviewers" will then

Table 3.1 The Basic Components of a Scientific Journal Article

Article Component	*Description*
Title	The title of a journal article will usually contain a description of the study variables, or what is being looked at. It will usually label the independent (IV) or predictive variable (the variable that you think is driving the association or difference) and the dependent or outcome variable (the variable that you think is being impacted by the IV). It might also mention a specific population being studied. For example, "Social Integration and Pulmonary Function in the Elderly" Crittenden et al. (2014) – Social integration is the predictor variable, pulmonary function is the outcome variable, and the population being looked at is the older people.
Abstract	The abstract is the brief summary that is provided for each article – this makes it easy for readers to see the main hypothesis and methods of the study, as well as the results and authors' conclusions. Thus, a reader can decide from the abstract whether what is being presented is relevant to them.
Introduction	Here is where the authors justify the importance of their research, and why the questions they are asking are worthy of study. They will usually present some background research and statistics and then present their guiding theory or framework. Usually, in the last paragraph of the introduction, you will find the authors' hypotheses/predictions.
Method	In the method section, you will find exactly how the research was conducted. It will explain the study design that was chosen (correlational, longitudinal, and experimental) Here, you will read about how study participants were recruited, and what the final sample looked like. There will be detailed descriptions of how all the variables were measured or manipulated, and how the study was set up.
Results	The results section is the most technical part of the paper. It will include what statistical tests were used to analyze and interpret the data. Not only will the results section be number-heavy, but it will also have numerous tables and figures to help display the data in a more understandable way.
Discussion	Also sometimes called the conclusion, the discussion section will reiterate the initial questions asked by the researchers and then summarize what was found in the results. The researchers will then draw bigger conclusions about theories and future directions. The authors will also discuss the strengths and weaknesses of the study.
References	The last section is the reference section, where you can find all the previous work that was referred to, for further exploration of the topic.

provide feedback and make a recommendation regarding next steps. These recommendations usually consist of a rejection of the paper, a "revise and resubmit," or an acceptance. Most often, the paper will go through several rounds of peer review. Once the peer reviewers have a consensus agreement that the paper is ready to publish, it is sent one last time to the editor, who has the final say.

It is through this process that we hope the best quality research gets published. Now, let's look at the type of research that gets published. We can divide up the research into a hierarchy of evidence – some research provides better evidence than others. Take a look at Figure 3.1, which discusses the hierarchy of medical

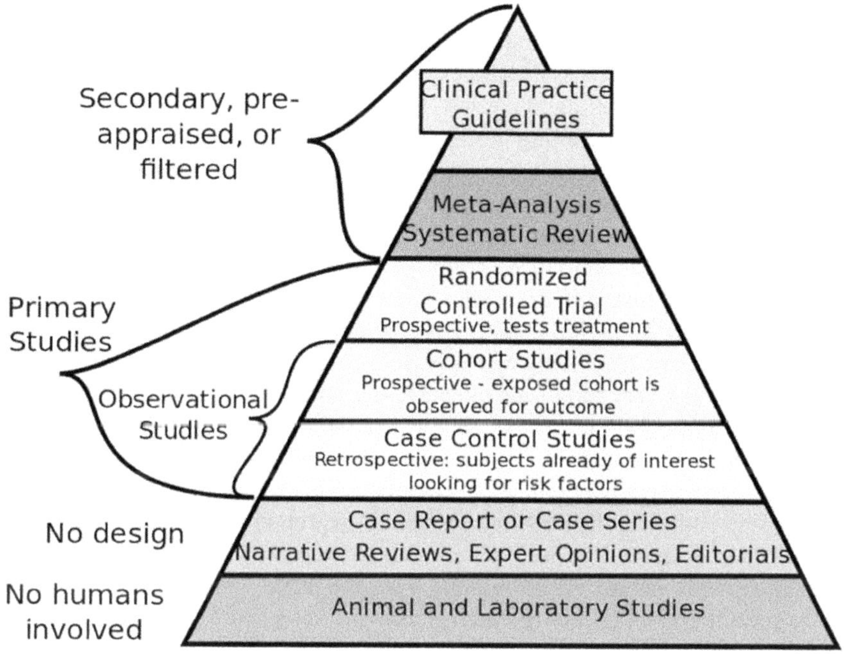

Figure 3.1 Hierarchy of Medical Research Publications.

research, which is what Louis Creed would be working with in his role as the director of university health services.

When it comes to evidence regarding human health outcomes, animal studies and in-vitro studies done in laboratories (think cells in a petri dish) provide us with basic knowledge, but in order to be useful, they need to be subject to further, human-centric research. Case studies, on the other hand, do use humans, but it is limited to just one, or a few, people. When Louis Creed presented his paper to the New England Conference on College and University Medicine, he presented a case study on "Henry Montez," the pseudonym he used for Victor Pascow. He received positive feedback, so from the case study, his next step may be to do a more planned out and intentional study on multiple people, as opposed to just one. We will discuss more about case studies later in this chapter when we talk about *The Dark Half.*

Leaving case, animal, and in-vitro studies behind, we now get into the realm of research designs. Case-control studies are when we collect data on things that have already happened. For example, we may look at people who have heart disease and those who do not have heart disease and ask them to think back to the type of career they had throughout most of their lives and the type of job stressors they faced.[1] We would then compare the differences in these retrospective reports between the groups to see what work factors might be associated with heart disease.

Since many people have a hard time accurately recalling the past, the next research design on the hierarchy is the cohort study – where we follow large groups of people over time, collecting data as we go, to see what is happening to them in real time, and how it impacts their health.

One issue with these types of studies, which are observational in nature, is that they have a hard time getting at causes. They can get at associations, but because so many things can be happening in someone's life at once, we might not be able to measure all of them, and conclusions will not be strong. What needs to happen for causal conclusions is that we have to test our hypotheses in more controlled environments and be able to compare groups of people in meaningful ways. This brings us to experiments and randomized controlled trials (RCTs). RCTs are considered the gold standard of research, especially when we are talking about treatment effectiveness.[2] We will discuss RCTs a bit more in the second half of this chapter when we discuss *The Dark Half* being an expressive writing endeavor by King.

However, at the very top of the evidence hierarchy are what we call secondary articles – these are journal articles that synthesize multiple primary studies (the case controls, cohorts, and RCTs mentioned above). When it comes to secondary articles, we have narrative reviews, systematic reviews, and meta-analyses. Narrative reviews synthesize the already published research in a casual, non-systematic way, and they are actually placed lower on the hierarchy because they can often be very subjective in nature. As is obvious from the name, systematic reviews have strict criteria for how primary research studies are searched for, included, and analyzed. And finally, at the very top, you have the meta-analysis – which not only follows the systematic review rules, but it also gathers all the data from those primary studies and reanalyzes them as a whole. This is done in hopes of reducing some of the biases that are inherent in research and allows us to get a clearer picture of the phenomena we are studying. When it comes to clinical professions, and what Louis Creed seeks out, we have clinical practice guidelines above meta-analyses and systematic reviews. These are actually called tertiary sources, and they are where all the information gathered within the pyramid is used to suggest treatments and describe exactly how they should be delivered. For example, after all the research had been conducted on how best to treat a massive head wound like the one suffered by Victor Pascow, the exact guidelines for how to do it would be published in a clinical practice publication.

When possible, in this paper, I try to present results from systematic reviews and meta-analyses – the top of the pyramid for health psychology research. When a systematic review or metanalysis has yet to be conducted, I try to stick to findings that have been reproduced in multiple primary papers. Other times, I may present data based on just one primary study because what they did was very cool, or very pertinent to the Stephen King material we are covering.

Box 3.2 The File Drawer Problem

As the legend has it, and as Stephen King himself has often explained, *Pet Sematary* was not meant to see the light of day (Breznican, 2019). The book is based on King's own experience living along a busy highway in Maine, while he had young kids, and those kids had pets. Unfortunately for his daughter, her cat Smucky fell victim to the busy highway, and became the inspiration for Ellie Creed's cat Church. After finishing the novel, King felt it was just too dark and upsetting, and he wound up hiding it away in a file drawer somewhere. It wasn't until he had to come up with a novel to hand over to Doubleday to meet a contractual obligation that *Pet Sematary* exited the drawer and entered our imaginations. It makes you wonder how many other great stories are hidden out there in people's file drawers, waiting to be told.

And this, in essence, is what we call in research the File Drawer Problem. In the late 1970s when *Pet Sematary* was presumably sitting in a file drawer, the psychologist Robert Rosenthal coined the term File Drawer Problem (Rosenthal, 1979). The problem presented here is that when it comes to research studies, there is a bias toward publishing the results when the researcher actually found something, not when they didn't find something. Within the research endeavor, studies can result with findings that are either (1) positive or significant – they show differences between groups, or that A is associated with be B, or causes B, and so forth. – or (2) null-or non-significant – they show no differences between groups, or that A is not associated with B, or does not cause B, and so forth. Publishers, funders, and all the people invested in research love positive and significant findings – we are getting somewhere! Thus, those studies with positive/significant results are more likely to get published or see the light of day. Those studies that have null findings are, in essence, sent to a $P > .05$ cemetery, and no one gets to see the associations and causes that don't exist.

Why is this problematic? We aren't getting the full story. What if ten different labs did a study on whether intelligence quotient (IQ) was associated with cortisol response to horror stories? One study found that people who had high IQs had less cortisol response to horror stories than those with lower IQs and concluded that people with higher IQs were not emotionally reactive to horror. But the other nine studies found that no such association existed. There were no IQ differences in how people respond to horror stories. According to the File Drawer Problem, that first study is the one that would get published, and the null results of the other nine would not be made known. Now it is out there that high IQ people are cold and callous and have no biological reaction when they see horrifying things happen. Yet nine other studies found that this was not the case, and so chances are the finding of the first study was an anomaly. Oh well, too bad. Off to the null findings cemetery you go!

The argument is that we need to end the bias of only publishing positive results. This will give everyone a better sense of what ALL the data are actually telling us, and it might also prevent time and money being spent on findings that are red herrings. Science has been trying to combat this bias for decades now. There have been journals started whose sole purpose is to publish only null results, but they have seen limited success (Kozlov, 2024). There is also a push to have journals accept pre-registered reports. That is, researchers would submit their study designs and hypotheses to a journal before data collection, and if accepted, the journal would publish the paper regardless of whether the findings were positive or null. Despite all of this, there is still a long way to go – and the null findings cemetery remains a popular place.

Conducting Research in Health Psychology – Let *The Dark Half* Light the Way

When I think about a person of science, and the scientific method, I think about Louis Creed and *Pet Sematary*. Yet when I think of the types of things that we want to study in health psychology, and the ways we go about doing it, I think about *The Dark Half* (see Box 3.3 for summary). One of the reasons is that for me, *The Dark Half* is a reactionary novel, and, in essence, health psychology is so much about our reaction to things – our biology reacting to our psychological and social world, and vice versa.

What do I mean when I say I think *The Dark Half* is a reactionary novel? I am referring to the fact that King wrote it in reaction to having his Richard Bachmann pseudonym outed by a bookstore clerk. If you don't know, Stephen King wrote several books under the pen name Richard Bachmann; these include *Rage*, *The Long Walk*, *Roadwork*, *The Running Man* (Chapter 6), *Thinner* (Chapter 4), *The Regulators*, and *Blaze*. From all that I have read, King was pretty perturbed by losing his alter ego, and the imagined horror that could have resulted plays out in *The Dark Half*.

Box 3.3 *The Dark Half*

King published *The Dark Half* in 1989, and it tells the story of a writer, Thad Beaumont. Thad, an English professor at the local university, has had little success with his highly intellectual and literary works. However, when he creates the pen name George Stark, and starts writing dark and decrepit novels about the psychopathic Alexis Machine, his writing career takes off.

Eventually, someone figures out that Thad is George and blackmails him to keep the secret. Instead of playing the blackmailer's game, Thad and his wife Elizabeth (they also have twin babies) decide to tell the world Thad's secret. In a publicity play, *People* magazine sets up a photo shoot where Thad and Elizabeth stand in front of George Stark's fake tombstone, smiling over the grave of Thad's alter ego, who was "Not a Very Nice Guy."

⚠ **[Spoiler Alert]** That fake grave gives birth to something more than a funny photo-op – emerging from the soil later that night is George Stark, and he is not happy that he has been killed off by Thad. He goes off killing people in Thad's town, as well as Thad's editor, agent, and the people involved in the photoshoot. Local law enforcement, including the beloved King character Alan Pangborn, immediately suspect Thad. Forensics taken at the crime scene also seem to support this – Thad's fingerprints are found all over, and they also find that Thad and George Stark have similar voice patterns. Yet Thad has some pretty tight alibis, and law enforcement starts to see him as a target, instead of the perpetrator.

Thad begins to notice that he may be psychically connected to George Stark. For example, he knows that George is driving around in a jacked-up Oldsmobile Toronado with a bumper sticker on the back that says, "HIGH-TONED SON OF A BITCH." He knows things about George, and George knows things about him. The fact that they have the same fingerprints, and the same voice patterns, and so forth, has both Thad and Alan Pangborn on edge.

Doing some slick detective work, Alan eventually finds out that as a boy, Thad was plagued by crippling headaches and seizures. What was believed to be a tumor that doctors successfully removed was actually Thad's unborn twin (the doctors left this part out of their diagnosis to Thad's parents). The questions asked then are – is George the ghost of Thad's unborn twin? Does Thad just have two personalities, one of which is his "twin" George? These are the questions that Alan and Thad care about, but there is a certain high-toned son of a bitch who doesn't care at all – he just wants to stay alive, but he is deteriorating rapidly. It seems that both George and Thad cannot exist as separate entities – and this fact leads to a showdown between the two. A showdown in which only one of them survives.

Case Studies – Low on the Hierarchy, but Important!

Case studies may be low on the data hierarchy, but they are extremely important in terms of foundational ideas in psychology. The most famous example of a case study that moved psychology forward, particularly in terms of our understanding of the brain and its "localization of function," is Phineas Gage. Localization of function refers to the fact that we know particular brain regions are specialized – for example, the back of the brain, or the occipital lobe is mostly responsible for all of our visual processing. We did not always have this understanding of the brain – for example, the philosopher René Descartes (him again!) just thought the brain was one large organ, and from that, scientists thought that all of our abilities were evenly distributed throughout. A fad in the early 19th century, called phrenology, started to get closer to the truth – it's creator, Franz Joseph Gall, insisted that it was bumps on our head that indicated areas of functional specification.

Ask any introductory psychology student and they should know Phineas Gage. His story has some Stephen King-esque body horror to it, so it easily sticks to one's mind and imagination.

In 1848, Phineas Gage, a socially adept, even-tempered, hardworking, and responsible railroad man, was working on a Vermont railroad line when disaster struck. He was preparing site for a rock blast, using a tamping iron (see Figure 3.2, with Phineas holding said tamping iron) to pack the needed explosive powder. Unfortunately for him, somewhere in the process, the tamping iron hit a rock, creating a spark that set off the explosive powder. The result? The explosion turned the tamping iron into a high-speed projectile that found its way through Gage's cheekbone, through his brain, and out the top of his head.

Amazingly enough, Gage survived, but he was "different." He was no longer able to navigate social situations appropriately – he became uninhibited and inappropriate around others. The once responsible Gage was no longer able to make plans and stick to them, or to make rational decisions. However, his speech, his ability to walk, and his memory were fully intact after the initial recovery. As a case study, this was a clear demonstration that all of our abilities were not equally dispersed throughout our brain, but that certain areas were the source of certain abilities. Where Phineas Gage experienced the damage, now called the frontal lobe, is understood to be the source of our higher order functioning – planning, logical

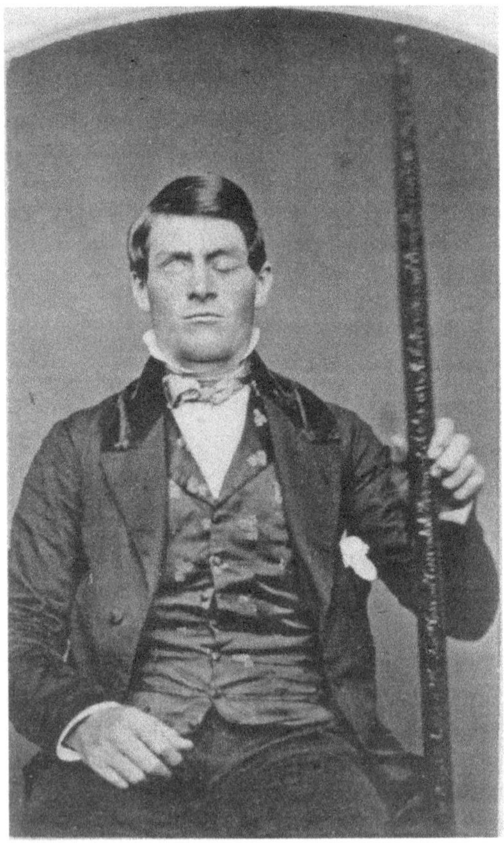

Figure 3.2 Phineas Gage and the Tamping Iron.

thinking, and personality. The accident did leave Gage with seizures, which were eventually the cause of his death 12 years after the accident.

Let's go back to *The Dark Half* – a good example of how case studies can come about. Poor 11-year-old Thad Beaumont, in the year 1960, begins experiencing some excruciating headaches. Initially dismissed by doctors as his nerves, and something he will just have to live with, a frightening episode involving a serious seizure leads to exploratory brain surgery. The doctors suspect a brain tumor, but what they find is so startling, and so rare, it enters case study territory.

⚠ **[Spoiler Alert]** As they open up Thad's skull, a nurse screams in horror, losing her mind and probably her job at the same time. The surgeon looks into the skull:

"Just incredible. This is really one for the books" (King, 2016, p.9).

The books he is referring to are medical journals, where he will probably write this up as a case study. What the doctor is going to write up is that when "Patient X's" skull was opened up – they saw a human eye, part of a nose, fingernails, and teeth. The surgeons are able to remove most of it, and are left to wonder – how? The answer – an absorbed twin. While that may be common (according to the doctor), having an absorbed twin that manifests itself in the brain of the pre-teen surviving twin – unheard of. Let's get it to press!!

Twin Studies

Of course, in *The Dark Half* – we have the "Twins" – George Stark and Thad Beaumont. In a sense – they are the same person genetically, but they have manifested themselves in very different ways through how they have developed across the life span. This, in essence, is the nature versus nurture debate framed in a horror context – how much are George and Thad the same because of their genetic makeup (the nature) and how much are they different because they experienced completely different upbringings and lives (the nurture)?

This brings up an important research method – not just in health psychology – but in many human-oriented sciences that ask questions about nature versus nurture. The method is referred to as the twin study, and it utilizes the fact that when it comes to twins, there are two types – monozygotic (MZ) and dizygotic (DZ).

The word zygote refers to an egg, so monozygotic refers to the fact that the twins develop from one egg. That one egg then divides itself into two different embryos that share 100% of their genetic makeup – for example, they are always the same sex, because their DNA is identical. Hence, they are referred to as identical twins. Dizygotic refers to the fact that there are two eggs, and they are then fertilized by two different sperm. Just like any siblings, they share about 50% of their DNA – they just happen to grow in the same womb at the same time. Dizygotic twins are what we are referring to when we say fraternal twins.

What does all this have to do with research? Quite a lot, actually. We can look at twins, follow them over time, and figure out a trait's heritability. Basically, how much of the differences between people are due to genetic variability, and how much is due to environmental factors.

Let's take this step by step to see how it works. First off, we need twins to study. There are many large twin studies out there that follow thousands of both MZ and

DZ twins. There is the Gemini Twin Research study, which has been following twins who were born in England and Wales in 2007 for almost two decades (Van Jaarsveld et al., 2010). Since the researchers here are taking a very specific population (twins born in 2007) and following them over time, we call this a cohort study (cohorts play an important part in health psychology – see Box 3.5 for other cohort studies you should know about). More specifically, this is a birth cohort study, because, of course, we have been following them since birth. In the United States, we have the Mid-Atlantic Twin Registry (MATR; Lilley et al., 2019), which consists of data on approximately 60,000 twins that have been followed for over 40 years. There is also Twins Research Australia (TRA; Murphy et al., 2019) and the Swedish Twin Registry (Zagai et al., 2019), to name a few more.

There are countless twin studies and registries around the world, and once we have the data, we can start to make some comparisons. Going back to our descriptions of twins, we have MZ twins, which share 100% of their DNA, and DZ twins, which share around 50%. Following these twins over time, and having them reared in the same environment, we can then ask some questions. We can look at something, let's say, that keeps in line with the themes of *The Dark Half*; we can look at the trait of psychopathy (of which George Stark, that high-toned son-of-a-bitch, has in spades). While what I am going to present here in terms of data is purely hypothetical, psychopathy itself is not. In our current understanding, we can divide psychopathy into its affective (aka emotional) components, its cognitive (aka thoughts) components, and its behavioral (aka actions) components (Gillespie et al., 2023). Emotionally, psychopathy consists of being unkind and lacking the emotions of guilt or remorse. In terms of thinking, manipulation and dominance are at the forefront, with irresponsibility and lack of inhibitions manifesting themselves behaviorally. These traits are unfortunately not just a work of fiction but are present in everyday life – according to a recent meta-analysis, approximately 4.5% of the general adult population has psychopathy (Sanz-García et al., 2021).

Now, we want to understand whether psychopathy stems from nature (genetics) or from nurture (developmental environmental influences). In essence – are you born into psychopathy, or is it made? Now, this is where we are getting into hypotheticals, just to show you how twin studies would go about answering this question. A classic twin study will assess psychopathy in both MZ and DZ twins, and figure out the correlation between the two.

Quick stop – what is a correlation? A correlation is just a calculation to see how well two variables relate to each other. In this case, you have two people, twins, and you rate the level of psychopathy (based on a measurement like the Hare Psychopathy checklist) (Hare, 1990). If the twins' scores are similar, we say that their scores are correlated. We would give the relationship between the scores a number, called the correlation coefficient. This number is between −1 and +1, with a 0 being indicative of no relationship.

Thus, after we measure levels of psychopathy in each twin, we do our correlations. If we find that MZ twins (the ones that share 100% of their DNA) have significantly more similar psychopathy scores than the DZ twins (only share about 50% DNA), then this is indicative of the psychopathy coming from genetic influence. If, on the other hand, we find that the MZ and DZ twins both have similarities in levels of psychopathy, we can say that it is probably due more to how they are being raised, as opposed to purely genetic influence.

With these data, we can calculate the index of heritability – or what percentage of psychopathy is due to genes. Look at the hypothetical data in Table 3.2. It compares two studies – one that shows differences between MZ and DZ twins, and the other shows no difference.

Study 1 indicates that psychopathy is highly heritable, or based on genetics, whereas study 2 has a much lower heritability rate. The data I made up in study 2 seem to be correct with what happened with Thad and George. Thad has a little bit of that "high-toned son-of-a-bitch" in him, but chances are, it was more about the environment he grew up in that led Thad to be who he is, compared to his "twin."

Why would knowing the heritability rate of traits and diseases be important to health psychology? As we discussed in Chapter 1, health psychology is attempting to use a biopsychosocial model to help prevent and treat illness. Health promotion, prevention, and treatment in this area can be done on modifiable factors – such as environmental impacts, and so forth. Knowing whether something is amenable to such intervention is hugely important. If something is highly genetically based, a biopsychosocial approach may not be as appropriate. For example, the things that we discuss in this book, like infectious disease, respiratory disease, high blood pressure, coronary heart disease, and major depressive disorder, have low heritability rates (Polubriaginof et al., 2018). This leaves more room for understanding how these diseases develop and maintain themselves, outside of genetic effects. Which is exactly what health psychology is trying to do!

Table 3.2 Hypothetical Heritability Rates for Psychopathy

Study	*MZ Correlation (Identical Twins)*	*DZ Correlation (Non-identical Twins)*	*Heritability*[a] *(MZ correlation – DZ correlation) × 2*
Study 1	0.78	0.36	0.84 (84%)
Study 2	0.47	0.32	0.30 (30%)

[a] This is Falconer's formula for heritability. You simply take the correlation of the trait among dizygotic twins and subtract it from the correlation of the trait in monozygotic twins, and then double the difference (Falconer, 1965).

Box 3.5 Important Health Psychology Longitudinal Cohort Studies

As mentioned in our discussion of twin studies – one way that we figure out what biopsychosocial factors influence people's health and wellbeing overtime is through longitudinal cohort studies. Longitudinal means that the data are collected over time, and the cohort means that we are following the same group of people. Some important cohorts within health psychology include:

Harvard Study of Adult Development – This was one of the very first cohort studies, and the longest running. The cohort consisted of men who had graduated from Harvard between the years of 1939 and 1944. This consisted of 268 men, including John F. Kennedy and Leonard Bernstein. As of 2017, 19 of the men were still with us (Fuchsman, 2023). The study has provided a wealth of information regarding what makes a healthy life – both physically and mentally. For example, analyzing this cohort, it was found that being pessimistic at age 25 led to more health problems later on in life. Pessimism here refers to habitually believing that bad things happen all the time (they are stable), in all things (they are global) and because of who you are (they are internal). Seeing the world in this way led to poor physical health later in life, regardless of your health at age 25 (Peterson et al., 1988).

Dunedin Study – The Dunedin Study started in New Zealand in the 1970s – it has followed people who were born in Dunedin, New Zealand, between 1972 and 1973 for over 50 years. At the start of the study, there were 1,037 participants (Poulton et al., 2023). One focus of the Dunedin study was mental health, particularly anxiety. By following this cohort since they were born, researchers could make strong connections between early life experiences and the development of phobias and anxiety disorders in early adulthood (Poulton et al., 2023). This may explain why watching Tim Curry as Pennywise on TV when I was 12 led to a very strong fear of white face close. If you know, you know!

Framingham Heart Study (FHS) – Recognizing the epidemiological shift from communicable diseases to non-communicable, the Framingham Heart Study began in 1948 in an attempt to better understand coronary heart disease. There have been multiple cohorts, consisting of approximately 15,000 people. We as a society are indebted to the FHS for how much it has taught us about cardiovascular health. For example, the data were used to show that anger and hostility are significant risk factors for atrial fibrillation, an irregular heart rhythm that can lead to heart failure (Eaker et al., 2004). These findings and others have significant implications for Bill Hodges, of King's *The Bill Hodges Trilogy* – which we will explore in Chapter 5.

The National Longitudinal Study of Adolescent to Adult Health (Add Health) – During the years 1994–1995, Add Health recruited approximately 20,000 students aged 12–19 for their cohort study (Harris et al., 2019). At first, the main goal was to look at the under-researched topic of adolescent health and wellbeing, but now that decades of data are available, it can be used to see how the experiences of adolescence impact adult health and wellbeing. Important findings stemming from the Add Health cohort include some interesting findings about how your friend's parents can influence your substance use when you are a teenager (Shakya et al., 2012) and how neighborhood disadvantage can lead to significant increases in the body mass index (Burdette & Needham, 2012).

Health and Retirement Study (HRS) – The HRS is a multidisciplinary cohort study that began in 1992 with the goal of studying the health and wellbeing of working and retired adults in the United States who were born between 1931 and 1941 (Fisher & Ryan, 2018). Important findings here include connections between changes in work expectations and depression and suicidal ideation (Mezuk et al., 2022), retirement with physical health (Clouston & Denier, 2017), and social integration with lung function (Crittenden et al., 2018).

Measuring the Fear – And Psychopathy

Now that we have talked about specific types of studies, let's briefly review how we go about measuring the variables that we are interested in looking at within those studies. Remember, variables are anything that varies, and we are interested in getting the most accurate measurement of that variation.

Let's use a hypothetical research question based on *The Dark Half*, to illustrate how this works. Throughout the novel, there are lots of descriptions of fear, and fear responses, especially among George Stark's victims. Based on the work of Walter Cannon and many others who followed him, we know, in general, how emotions (fear in particular) manifest themselves in our biology (remember HPA and SAM axes?). But let's say our question takes it a step further – how does emotion manifest itself physically in someone like George Stark? And by George Stark, I mean someone high in trait psychopathy, as we discussed earlier. The research question is – When someone experiences fear, how does their level of psychopathy influence their biological reactions to the fear?

In essence, our research question is focused on three variables – the first one is our independent variable (IV) – the one we think is causing something else to happen. Our IV here is the experience of fear. The dependent variable (DV), the one we think is being impacted by the IV, is biological reactions. The third variable is what we would call a moderating variable – a variable we think will lessen or increase the strength of the relationship between the IV and DV. Here, the moderator is psychopathy.

In order to test this, we need to measure the variables. For the IV here, I can either measure someone's level or fear, or I can manipulate it experimentally. I could do an experiment (described more in the next section) where I randomly assign study participants to a fearful condition (watching Stephen King's *It*,[3] let's say) or a non-fearful condition (watching Pixar's *Up*) and then we see the differences in their biological reactions.

Since this section is all about measuring variables, we are not going to do the randomized control experiment; instead, we are going to look at the data cross-sectionally – collect all the data at once and see how they are associated. However, there is one thing I need to make sure I do, and that is to get everyone in a fear state. So, I am going to expose everyone to Stephen King's *It*, just to make sure everyone is good and scared. This is quasi-manipulation on my part.

Okay, so we have everyone watching *It,* and now we want to measure how much fear they are actually experiencing. We can measure the IV in several ways. We can observe the participants and have a set of criteria that we will use to code whether we think they are feeling fear. Do they cover their eyes? Do they scream? Do they jump out of their chairs? There could be any number of behaviors that we could observe that we could then use to measure their level of fear. Usually, when we do behavioral measurements like this, we have at least two people watching, and those two people must agree on what they are seeing. We call this inter-rater reliability.

Observations are one way to measure the variable, but they can be time-consuming, and they are open to several forms of bias – such as people changing the way they behave because they are being watched. Instead, we might consider doing self-report. Here, we just ask people if they are afraid. We could create our own series of questions, or we could use questionnaires that have already been shown to be valid (accurate) and reliable (consistent) measures of fear. We could use a measurement like the Profile of Mood States (POMS; McNair, 1992) or the Positive and Negative Affect Schedule (PANAS; Watson et al., 1988), which ask about fear in addition to other emotions, or something more specific like the Fear Questionnaire (FQ; Marks & Mathews, 1979).

We could do the same thing when we go to measure the level of psychopathy. We could absolutely do an observational measurement, and maybe we want to include some documentation analysis – like how many times have they been arrested? How many times were they in trouble growing up for antisocial or conduct issues? But it may be that we are looking at a "community sample" – that is, people who may have variable levels of psychopathy, but they aren't considered to have the clinically significant behaviors an observational measure would pick up. In that case, we would want to consider self-report.

If we are going to go the self-report route, we will want to collect these data BEFORE they start watching *It*, so that our quasi-manipulation doesn't impact their answers. We have already mentioned Hare's (1990) psychopathy checklist, but there are others to choose from, like the Self-Report Psychopathy Scale (Levenson et al., 1995). Once we pick out which self-report measure we want to use, we will then give it to the subjects prior to them watching the movie. Since we are measuring psychopathy here, which has a huge amount of stigma associated with it, we want to make sure we let the participants know that their answers are anonymous – we collect the data with subject numbers instead of names. This anonymity helps reduce social desirability bias, which is basically when people "fake good."

Lastly, we want to see the biological ramifications of being afraid (and whether psychopathy moderates the relationship), so we need to collect some biological, or psychophysiological, data. This is where health psychology is truly indebted to Walter Cannon, as he was the first to use things like heart rate, blood pressure, metabolism, and adrenaline levels, to investigate emotions. What are some of the common biological measures we might use today to assess our DV and answer our research questions?

We could look at how fear impacts one's cardiovascular system, by looking at things like heart rate, blood pressure, or heart rate variability. We could look at different hormone markers like cortisol, testosterone, or oxytocin. Mostly, when we are interested in whether or not a threat has been perceived, and stress has been experienced, we look at cortisol. The nice thing about cortisol is that you can look at it via saliva, so it is not as invasive. If you want to look at long-term exposure to stress, you can even look at cortisol via hair samples!

We could also look at other things that are indicative of biological responses – like pupil dilation (our pupils get bigger when we are feeling threatened) or skin conductance response (which we discussed in Chapter 1). If we are interested in whether the body is becoming more inflamed, we could look at some immune markers that are indicative of inflammation – like c-reactive protein or interleukin-6 (IL-6). Amazingly, this is just a small portion of the biological measurements we use in health psychology (though they are the most widely used). We have really come a long way since Walter Cannon!

Once we have gathered all of the data, we go and get our friend John the statistician, and he figures out (1) is there a relationship between one's level of fear and their biology? And (2) does the level of psychopathy reported moderate this relationship? And then it is time for the conference, the peer review, and the glory (or the file drawer).

Intervention – The Dark Half ***as Expressive Writing and RCTs***

We have been dropping the concept of RCTs here and there, but now it is time for a health psychology/Stephen King example. For this, we are going to go back to expressive writing. If you remember, expressive writing was a way to turn the "talking cure" into the "writing" cure – by having people write about their traumas, stressors, and emotions, in order to improve their physical and mental health (Pennebaker & Chung, 2013).

Expressive writing overlaps with *The Dark Half* in two distinct ways. One is that *The Dark Half* could be another instance of Stephen King working out his demons on the page. In this case, the demons may be the guy who outed him as Richard Bachman, and maybe the death of Richard Bachman himself and what that meant for King's writing in the future. A lot to process there! Then of course we have Thad Beaumont, who has to literally write out the demons to save his life (with a Berol Black Beauty pencil).

When doing our RCT, we start with our population of interest – here we are going to say we are interested in people who have had their writing alias die of cancer (the diagnosis given to Richard Bachman by King). Just imagine that there are thousands of writers out there who have lost their pseudonyms and they need to work through some stuff (this is the technical therapeutic term).

Yes, there are thousands afflicted, but we can't study them all (we do not have the time or the money), so we randomly recruit 100 to be in our study. Once we provide them with informed consent and they have agreed to be in the study, we will randomly assign them (to ensure there is no selection bias) to one of two conditions: (1) the expressive writing condition where they write about a trauma that has occurred in their life, and the emotions around it, or (2) a control condition where they write about something fairly neutral, like their plans for the day or what they ate for breakfast (Smyth, 1998). The subjects are asked to do this over several days and several sessions, and the researchers collect the health and wellbeing measurements of interest.

At the end of the study, the researchers will compare the 50 people in the expressive writing condition to the 50 people in the controlled writing condition, to see if there are any differences in their health and wellbeing. While we don't have data on what the results would look like among our sample of tortured writers, we do have a plethora of data showing significant differences in outcomes between the two groups in other populations (Smyth & Helm, 2003).

One biological measure we have not talked about yet is wound healing. Researchers will perform punch biopsies (a 4 mm skin puncture) on healthy subjects and then see how long it takes their body to heal the wound. This is an excellent measure of how the immune system is functioning out in the real world, as opposed to a petri dish. In one study, participants were randomly assigned to either the expressive writing condition or the control condition and then given punch biopsies. What they found was that those in the expressive writing condition had greater healing of the wound 11 days later than those in the control condition (Koschwanez et al., 2013). This impact on wound healing has been replicated (Robinson et al., 2017), which indicates there is some way the expressive writing helps the immune system perform its day-to-day operations.

In a very brief nutshell, that is an example of how an RCT may be used in health psychology research. The RCT is truly the best way to get at the causal factor between IVs and DVs because it is assumed that the only difference between the two groups is the IV you are manipulating – here it is whether you write about trauma or breakfast. If the only thing different between the two groups is the type of writing and then there are significant differences in health (like wound healing) after the manipulation, it is assumed that the manipulation was what caused the changes. Unfortunately, we can't use RCT to answer all of our questions – as some variables just can't be manipulated, or it would be unethical for us to manipulate them. For example, if I am interested in how the generation you were born into affects your eating habits, I can't randomly assign you to be a Gen Zer, or a Millennial (these are called person variables, and they cannot be manipulated). On the other hand, if I am interested in how adverse childhood experiences impact immune function, it would be unethical for me to randomly assign some babies to have adverse experiences and some babies not to. That is why we have both the RCTs, and the correlational and longitudinal designs, as discussed in this chapter.

Versions of *Pet Sematary*

Novel: King, S. (1983). *Pet Sematary*. Doubleday.
Films:

Lambert, M. (Director). (1989). *Pet Sematary* [Film]. Paramount Pictures.
Lambert, M. (Director). (1992). *Pet Sematary Two* [Film]. Paramount Pictures.
Kölsch, K., & Widmyer, D. (Directors). (2019). *Pet Sematary* [Film]. Di Bonaventura Pictures; Room 101, Inc.; Paramount Pictures.
Beer, L. A. (Director). (2023). *Pet Sematary: Bloodlines* [Film]. Paramount Players; Di Bonaventura Pictures.

Audiobook (Audible Edition): King, S. (2018). *Pet Sematary* [Audiobook]. Simon & Schuster Audio. (Original work published 1983)[4]

Versions of *The Dark Half*

Novel: King, S. (1989). *The Dark Half*. Viking.
Film: Romero, G. A. (Director). (1993). *The Dark Half* [Film]. Dark Half Productions; Orion Pictures.
Audiobook: King, S. (2016). *The Dark Half* [Audiobook]. Simon & Schuster Audio. (Original work published 1989)

Further Exploration Questions

1 One of the reasons for using the systematic and regimented research methods described above is to combat confirmation bias. Confirmation bias is an error in thinking we often make – where we only pursue or look at the evidence around us that agrees with our ideas (see Nickerson, 1998, for an interesting review). That is, we only see, and only give credence to, things around us that support our view. The methods of science are meant to make a more impartial and unbiased collection of data. Throughout the works of Stephen King – you constantly see characters with strong confirmation bias. This is true of both *Pet Sematary* and *The Dark Half*, among countless others. Find distinct examples of confirmation bias in any Stephen King work – and then explain how using one of the methods or approaches discussed in this chapter could help combat the bias and ultimately get to the truth of the matter.
2 We asked the question in this chapter whether levels of fear influence certain biological outcomes, and whether psychopathy moderates this relationship. Based on the character of George Stark – what do you think? Do you think George Stark (high psychopathy) has the same biological reactions to fear as we (hopefully low psychopathy) do? Pick a biological outcome of interest to you (cortisol, blood pressure, IL-6, etc.) and then try to find the answer based on research that has already been published. Chances are it will be easy for you to find the fear connection, but what about the psychopathy part of the puzzle? Can you find anything relevant that would help inform a working hypothesis?

Notes

1 We will discuss health and occupational stress in more detail in Chapter 5, which explores the Bill Hodges trilogy.
2 RCTs are discussed in greater detail in Chapter 4, which covers placebo effects.
3 In my fake study scenario, they are watching the 1990 miniseries with Tim Curry as Pennywise – because, for me, he is one of the greatest elicitors of fear I can think of. No offense to Bill Skarsgård.
4 This Audible version of *Pet Sematary* is read by Michael C. Hall, who is known for playing serial killer Dexter Morgan in the TV show *Dexter*. He does an amazing job, and I highly recommend his narration. Just don't listen to it in your Jeep late at night while driving through central Pennsylvania. Your HPA axis can't handle that!

Bibliography

Ajzen, I. (1991). The theory of planned behavior. *Organizational Behavior and Human Decision Processes*, *50*(2), 179–211.

Andersson, C., Johnson, A. D., Benjamin, E. J., Levy, D., & Vasan, R. S. (2019). 70-year legacy of the Framingham heart study. *Nature Reviews Cardiology*, *16*(11), 687–698. https://doi.org/10.1038/s41569-019-0202-5

Bandura, A. (2013). Health promotion from the perspective of social cognitive theory. In C. Abraham, P. Norman, & M. Conner (Eds.), *Understanding and changing health behaviour: From health beliefs to self-regulation* (pp. 299–339).

Breznican, A. (2019, March 29). *Pet Sematary*: Stephen King on his most disturbing book. *Entertainment Weekly*. https://ew.com/movies/2019/03/29/pet-sematary-stephen-king-interview/

Burdette, A. M., & Needham, B. L. (2012). Neighborhood environment and body mass index trajectories from adolescence to adulthood. *Journal of Adolescent Health*, *50*(1), 30–37. https://doi.org/10.1016/j.jadohealth.2011.03.009

Clouston, S. A., & Denier, N. (2017). Mental retirement and health selection: Analyses from the US health and retirement study. *Social Science & Medicine*, *178*, 78–86. https://doi.org/10.1016/j.socscimed.2017.01.019

Crittenden, C. N., Murphy, M. L., & Cohen, S. (2018). Social integration and age-related decline in lung function. *Health Psychology*, *37*(5), 472. https://doi.org/10.1037/hea0000592

Crittenden, C. N., Pressman, S. D., Cohen, S., Janicki-Deverts, D., Smith, B. W., & Seeman, T. E. (2014). Social integration and pulmonary function in the elderly. *Health Psychology*, *33*(6), 535. https://doi.org/10.1037/hea0000029

Eaker, E. D., Sullivan, L. M., Kelly-Hayes, M., D'Agostino Sr, R. B., & Benjamin, E. J. (2004). Anger and hostility predict the development of atrial fibrillation in men in the Framingham offspring study. *Circulation*, *109*(10), 1267–1271. https://doi.org/10.1161/01.cir.0000118535.15205.8f

Falconer, D. S. (1965). The inheritance of liability to certain diseases, estimated from the incidence among relatives. *Annals of Human Genetics*, *29*(1), 51–76. https://doi.org/10.1111/j.1469-1809.1965.tb00500.x

Fisher, G. G., & Ryan, L. H. (2018). Overview of the health and retirement study and introduction to the special issue. *Work, Aging and Retirement*, *4*(1), 1–9. https://doi.org/10.1093/workar/wax032

Fuchsman, K. E. N. (2023). Harvard grant study of adult development: 1938–2022. *Journal of Psychohistory*, *51*(1), 27–44.

Gillespie, S. M., Jones, A., & Garofalo, C. (2023). Psychopathy and dangerousness: An umbrella review and meta-analysis. *Clinical Psychology Review*, *100*, 102240. https://doi.org/10.1016/j.cpr.2022.102240

Hare, R. D., Harpur, T. J., Hakstian, A. R., Forth, A. E., Hart, S. D., & Newman, J. P. (1990). The revised Psychopathy Checklist: Reliability and factor structure. *Psychological Assessment: A Journal of Consulting and Clinical Psychology*, *2*(3), 338–341.

Harris, K. M., Halpern, C. T., Whitsel, E. A., Hussey, J. M., Killeya-Jones, L. A., Tabor, J., & Dean, S. C. (2019). Cohort profile: The national longitudinal study of adolescent to adult health (add health). *International Journal of Epidemiology*, *48*(5), 1415–1415k. https://doi.org/10.1093/ije/dyz115

King, S. (2014). *Pet Sematary* (Kindle ed.). Scribnerhttps://www.amazon.com/Pet-Sematary-Stephen-King-ebook/dp/B00K3NEE56

King, S. (2016). *The Dark Half*. Scribner. https://www.amazon.com/Dark-Half-Stephen-King-ebook/dp/B018ER7L7U

Koschwanez, H. E., Kerse, N., Darragh, M., Jarrett, P., Booth, R. J., & Broadbent, E. (2013). Expressive writing and wound healing in older adults: A randomized controlled trial. *Psychosomatic Medicine*, *75*(6), 581–590. https://doi.org/10.1097/PSY.0b013e31829b7b2e

Kozlov, M. (2024). So you got a null result. Will anyone publish it? *Nature*, *631*(8022), 728–730. https://doi.org/10.1038/d41586-024-02383-9

Levenson, M. R., Kiehl, K. A., & Fitzpatrick, C. M. (1995). Assessing psychopathic attributes in a noninstitutionalized population. *Journal of Personality and Social Psychology*, *68*(1), 151. https://doi.org/10.1037/0022-3514.68.1.151

Lilley, E. C., Morris, A. T., & Silberg, J. L. (2019). The mid-atlantic twin registry of Virginia Commonwealth University. *Twin Research and Human Genetics*, *22*(6), 753–756. https://doi.org/10.1017/thg.2019.87

Marks, I. M., & Mathews, A. M. (1979). Brief standard self-rating for phobic patients. *Behaviour Research and Therapy*, *17*(3), 263–267.

McNair, D. M. (1992). *Profile of mood states*. Educational and Industrial Testing Service. https://doi.org/10.1037/t05057-000

Meyer, I. H. (2003). Prejudice, social stress, and mental health in lesbian, gay, and bisexual populations: Conceptual issues and research evidence. *Psychological Bulletin*, *129*(5), 674. https://doi.org/10.1037/0033-2909.129.5.674

Mezuk, B., Dang, L., Jurgens, D., & Smith, J. (2022). Work expectations, depressive symptoms, and passive suicidal ideation among older adults: Evidence from the health and retirement study. *The Gerontologist*, *62*(10), 1454–1465. https://doi.org/10.1093/geront/gnac110

Murphy, K., Lam, J., Cutler, T., Tyler, J., Calais-Ferreira, L., Li, S., … & Hopper, J. L. (2019). Twins research Australia: A new paradigm for driving twin research. *Twin Research and Human Genetics*, *22*(6), 438–445. https://doi.org/10.1017/thg.2019.101

Nickerson, R. S. (1998). Confirmation bias: A ubiquitous phenomenon in many guises. *Review of General Psychology*, *2*(2), 175–220. https://doi.org/10.1037/1089-2680.2.2.175

Pennebaker, J. W., & Chung, C. K. (2013). Expressive writing: Connections physical and mental health to Health. In H.S. Friedman (Ed.), *The Oxford handbook of health psychology*, (pp. 417–437). https://doi.org/10.1093/oxfordhb/9780195342819.013.0018

Peterson, C., Seligman, M. E., & Vaillant, G. E. (1988). Pessimistic explanatory style is a risk factor for physical illness: A thirty-five-year longitudinal study. *Journal of Personality and Social Psychology*, *55*(1), 23. https://doi.org/10.1037/0022-3514.55.1.23

Polubriaginof, F. C. G., Vanguri, R., Quinnies, K., Belbin, G. M., Yahi, A., Salmasian, H., … & Tatonetti, N. P. (2018). Disease heritability inferred from familial relationships reported in medical records. *Cell, 173*(7), 1692–1704.e11. https://doi.org/10.1016/j.cell.2018.04.032

Poulton, R., Caspi, A., & Moffitt, T. E. (2023). Fear and anxiety: Lessons learned from the Dunedin longitudinal study. *Neuroscience & Biobehavioral Reviews, 148*, 105118. https://doi.org/10.1016/j.neubiorev.2023.105118

Poulton, R., Guiney, H., Ramrakha, S., & Moffitt, T. E. (2023). The Dunedin study after half a century: Reflections on the past, and course for the future. *Journal of the Royal Society of New Zealand, 53*(4), 446–465. https://doi.org/10.1080/03036758.2022.2114508

Robinson, H., Jarrett, P., Vedhara, K., & Broadbent, E. (2017). The effects of expressive writing before or after punch biopsy on wound healing. *Brain, Behavior, and Immunity, 61*, 217–227. https://doi.org/10.1016/j.bbi.2016.12.015

Rosenthal, R. (1979). The file drawer problem and tolerance for null results. *Psychological Bulletin, 86*(3), 638. https://doi.org/10.1037/0033-2909.86.3.638

Sanz-García, A., Gesteira, C., Sanz, J., & García-Vera, M. P. (2021). Prevalence of psychopathy in the general adult population: A systematic review and meta-analysis. *Frontiers in Psychology, 12*, 661044. https://doi.org/10.3389/fpsyg.2021.661044

Shakya, H. B., Christakis, N. A., & Fowler, J. H. (2012). Parental influence on substance use in adolescent social networks. *Archives of Pediatrics & Adolescent Medicine, 166*(12), 1132–1139. https://doi.org/10.1001/archpediatrics.2012.1372

Smyth, J., & Helm, R. (2003). Focused expressive writing as self-help for stress and trauma. *Journal of Clinical Psychology, 59*(2), 227–235. https://doi.org/10.1002/jclp.10144

Smyth, J. M. (1998). Written emotional expression: Effect sizes, outcome types, and moderating variables. *Journal of Consulting and Clinical Psychology, 66*(1), 174. https://doi.org/10.1037/0022-006X.66.1.174

Van Jaarsveld, C. H., Johnson, L., Llewellyn, C., & Wardle, J. (2010). Gemini: A UK twin birth cohort with a focus on early childhood weight trajectories, appetite and the family environment. *Twin Research and Human Genetics, 13*(1), 72–78. https://doi.org/10.1375/twin.13.1.72

Watson, D., Clark, L. A., & Tellegen, A. (1988). Development and validation of brief measures of positive and negative affect: The PANAS scales. *Journal of Personality and Social Psychology, 54*(6), 1063. https://doi.org/10.1037/0022-3514.54.6.1063

Zagai, U., Lichtenstein, P., Pedersen, N. L., & Magnusson, P. K. (2019). The Swedish twin registry: Content and management as a research infrastructure. *Twin Research and Human Genetics, 22*(6), 672–680. https://doi.org/10.1017/thg.2019.99

4 Believing the Unbelievable

Placebos and Voodoo Curses

Believing the Unbelievable

There is no better example of our mind getting under our skin than placebo/nocebo effects. In the Stephen King cannon, you can find these effects throughout, but the most compelling and clear examples can be found in *It*, *Holly*, and *Thinner*.

Placebo and nocebo effects create quite a conundrum for those who follow the biomedical model. As you will see, there is no better example of how the mind and body interact than these effects. They are so important that they are a key part of medical research and "Gold Standard" clinical trials. Placebos are one of the rare cases where even the most hardened of biomedical practitioners must acknowledge the mind – body connection.

I may be getting ahead of myself here. Let's take a step back and go over what we actually mean by placebo/nocebo effects. Coming from Latin, placebo means "I shall please" and nocebo means "I shall harm." We give the name placebo or nocebo to treatments that have no active ingredients, or to those that, in and of themselves, would not be expected to change anything. In the case of placebo – we give someone a non-active treatment, and they feel better, and in the case of nocebo, they feel worse. The classic example is a sugar pill. If I give someone who has a headache a sugar pill, tell them that it is headache medicine, and they take it and their headache gets better, then we have a placebo effect. If I give someone a sugar pill and tell them it often gives people a rash, and lo and behold, they get a rash – that is the nocebo effect.

Why Are Placebo Effects Important?

There are many variables to think about when investigating the mechanism of how these effects work. How much does the person want to believe? Who is the one who gives them the treatment? How invasive is the treatment? We will talk about these as we explore the effects in Stephen King's works. For now, the most important thing to know is that in general, placebo effects can make up as much as 54% of a treatment's effectiveness (Hafliðadóttir et al., 2021) In other words, it could be that even with an active treatment, 54% of the improvement is due just to the patient expecting it to work as opposed to the aspects of the treatment itself.

DOI: 10.4324/9781003495994-4

Let's revisit that. I stated at the beginning that placebos play a key part in medical research, and they are a required component for gold standard clinical trials. If 54% of someone's improvement when placed on a medication is simply due to them expecting to get better, then how much is due to the actual medication that is given? That is what clinical researchers must find out. In most medical trials, there will likely be three conditions – some people will get no treatment, some will get a placebo treatment, and some will get the actual medication. Let's stick with the idea of headaches when illustrating this.

A researcher has come up with a new medicine to treat mild to moderate migraine headaches. To make sure it is the actual medicine that is working, the research group will recruit participants who experience mild to moderate migraine headaches and randomly assign them to the condition. About ⅓ of the participants will be placed into a "no treatment" group, where they will just come into the office, learn about the study and their condition, and understand how to monitor their migraine headaches for the next month. Another ⅓ will be randomly assigned to the placebo condition, where they will be given a bottle full of sugar pills that look just like the real medicine. They will be prescribed to take it the same way as the other ⅓ who are randomly assigned the actual medication.

One important thing to note – the study participants should not know what they are getting. You do not tell the ones getting no treatment that they are in the no treatment group, you do not tell the placebo group they are getting a placebo, and you do not tell the medication group that they are getting medication. This is called a blind study – the participants are blind to what their group is. This helps control for expectancy effects. Even better is the double-blind study. This is when the researcher, or the people collecting the data, don't know what condition the participants are in either. Usually, there is a group of data managers or a Data Safety Monitoring Board that knows the condition assignment, but the researchers on the ground do not. Having a double-blinded study goes a long way to reducing participant and observer bias, and increasing the credibility of the study.

Now back to our migraine medication study. About a month later, the study participants return, and they hand in their questionnaires about the amount and severity of migraines they have experienced since being enrolled in the clinical trial. If the medicine does work, we should see results similar to those shown in Figure 4.1.

In the "No Treatment" group, we see that there was a reduction in migraine symptoms by about 5%. This can be due to many things, including the participants getting better over the course of time, or just benefiting psychologically from being in a study and interacting with a doctor. In the "Placebo" group, we see a 32% reduction in migraine symptoms over the month. If we take out the 5% that is due to just time and being in the doctor's office, we would say that 27% of the improvement in symptoms is due to the placebo effect. This 27% reduction may be because the expectation is that they are taking the medicine and that they will improve because of it, and then they do. In the "Actual Medicine" group, we see a 64% reduction in migraine symptoms. If we take out the improvement due to time (5%) and the improvement due to placebo expectations (27%), then the study shows that 32% of the reduction was actually due to the medication, and no other

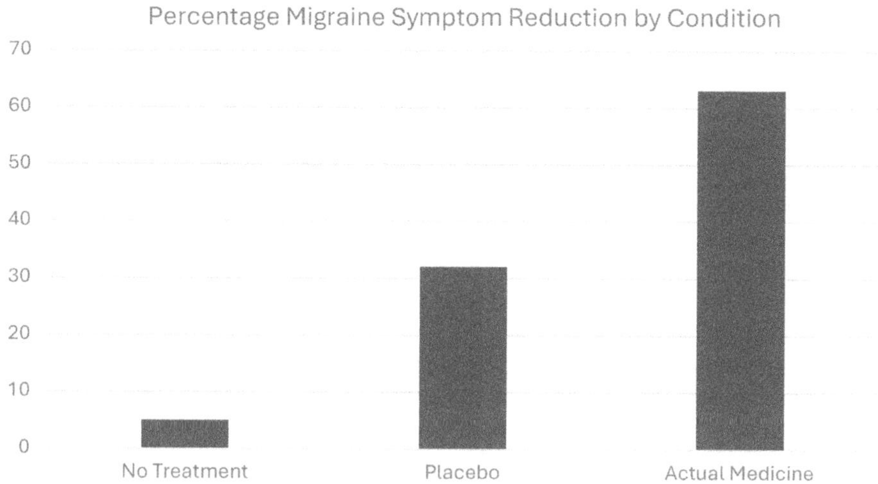

Figure 4.1 Treatment Effects for a Randomized, Double-Blind Three-Arm Trial of Migraine Medication.

factors. That is actually really good! This medicine is working above and beyond the healing benefits of time and placebo.

Thus, the gold standard for finding out whether your treatment actually works is including at least a placebo arm. But by including this, does that mean the biomedical community accepts that the mind plays a role in our physical functioning? Unfortunately, not likely. But you know who accepts this idea, and the power of placebo and nocebo effects? Yes, you guessed it – Stephen King! So, let's explore more about what we know about placebo and nocebo with characters from *It*, *Holly*, and *Thinner*.

The Real Horror Is the Placebo Effect – *Holly*

While I was reading *Holly* (see Box 4.1 for summary) for the first time, my husband asked me "how's the new Stephen King?" and I replied, "Well, the real horror here is the placebo effect!" That really stuck with me and, along with my *The Shining* experience, got this book to begin percolating in my head.

Box 4.1 *Holly*

While *Holly* is a great novel in and of itself, Holly Gibney is a character who is first introduced in Book 1 of the Bill Hodges trilogy *Mr. Mercedes* (Bill is the main focus of the next chapter in this book). She becomes an even more integral part of King's universe in Book 2, *Finders Keepers,* and Book 3, *End of Watch.* She is also a character in King's 2018 book *The Outsider* and is the main character in the 2020 short story "If It Bleeds." Then, in 2023, King published *Holly* – in which Holly takes more of a front stage role. Thus, if you choose to read *Holly* first, there may be many references to the previous works that may go over your head. Yet it is still an excellent read.

When *Holly* begins, we see that Holly is still an investigator for "Finders Keepers," the investigative agency that was founded by the now deceased Bill Hodges. Holly's current investigative partner, Pete Huntley, is down for the count with Covid-19, and Holly's unvaccinated mother has just succumbed to the disease. Taking on new clients is not on her priority list, but a desperate call from a mother looking for her missing 20-something daughter has Holly on the case.

⚠ **[Spoiler Alert]** The missing woman, Bonnie Dahl, ends up being one of many people missing from in and around the local college. Jorge Castro, an English professor, was thought to have left town of his own volition many years ago, yet no one – not even his family – ever heard from him again. Peter Steinmen, a young boy from town, Ellen Craslow, a janitor at the college, and Cary Dressler, an employee at the local bowling alley, all go missing as well.

While Holly is out investigating Bonnie Dahl's disappearance, and picking up on the other disappearances as well, we are introduced to the Professors Emily and Rodney Harris – who have had dealings with all of the missing persons. Emily Harris is a retired professor of English Literature, and Rodney is a retired professor of Life Sciences, both from the local college. Getting old has been hard on the Harrises – Emily has a crippling case of sciatica, and not only is Rodney suffering from arthritis, but he is also quickly slipping away from Alzheimer's disease.

Luckily for the couple, Rodney has spent his career in the Life Sciences as a top biologist and nutritionist, and he knows what will heal them – meat. What we come to find out is that it is not just any meat that provides the ultimate treatment for sciatica and Alzheimer's disease, but it is human meat that is required. Rodney has been doing "research" on this for years, and he has found a way to utilize almost every part of the human body for medicinal purposes. Yes, the missing people have been taken by the Harrises, prepped in their basement dungeon, and then refined into the food, creams, and medicines that the Harrises believe are keeping them alive.

Holly, being the intrepid investigator that she is, eventually connects all the missing (and dead) persons to the professors, but winds up being a prisoner herself in their meat prep prison. What happens to Holly and the old cannibals…will be up to you to read about at the end of *Holly*.

The Placebo Is People

Before we begin this discussion of the placebo effect in *Holly*, we must set the record straight. We will be working under the assumption that there are no medicinal qualities to human flesh, and that it can actually negatively impact your health (prion disease, anyone?). Therefore, what was happening to the professors when they improved was a placebo effect. ⚠ **[Spoiler Alert]** Holly tries to weaponize this fact, and she fights her captors in the basement: "It was the placebo effect all along, Emily. Expectation aids body chemistry" (King, 2023, p.404).

Holly is shocked that two seemingly intelligent professors could actually kill people and eat them because they think it is curing their ills. But human flesh as a placebo, and the context in which the "medicine" comes to them, has some pretty strong impacts on what a person is willing to believe and expect.

Who Was Prescribing the Placebo?

Rodney Harris is described as a stellar researcher and nutritionist, particularly in his early years. He was also known to be a difficult lecturer, which probably means he didn't (or couldn't) explain the material on a more basic level. We would call this the expert blind spot, and of course, it happens when someone is an expert in their field. It is also probably the case that he was very opinionated in terms of his expertise – that is, he was VERY confident in his knowledge, research, and the conclusions he drew from them. This means that with him delivering the placebo interventions, his wife was much more likely to expect that it would work, and then that expectation would lead to it actually working. Researchers hypothesize that the social context in which the placebo is delivered impacts how effective it is. In one study, when a physician delivered an inactive anti-allergy cream to participants (after they had been exposed to an allergy skin prick), those who considered the physician as having high competence and high warmth had significantly less of an allergic reaction than those who considered the physician as being incompetent and cold (Howe et al., 2017). It is clear that Rodney and his wife thought of him as competent, and that he was warm to her when giving her his human-based concoctions, so this probably increased how effective it was for her sciatica.

He may also be lecturing her on the WHY of how it works, and we know that when placebos are presented with descriptions of how and why they are going to work, they are more effective (Colloca & Miller, 2011). It may also be the case that along with the verbal cues, she did actually feel better (for some other reason, like just a natural fluctuation) and now she has associated the verbal instructions of her professor husband with the naturally occurring improvement, making future placebo effects that much stronger.

What Condition Was the Placebo Treating?

Both Rodney and Emily claim that eating human flesh keeps their pain at bay. For Emily, it is for her sciatica – which is actually a symptom, not a diagnosis (Valat et al., 2010). When someone says they are suffering from sciatica, they are referring to inflammation that causes compression of the nerves in the lower parts of the body. It can be very painful, with the feeling of pain starting in your lower back and then traveling down your legs. There aren't very many things that can be done for sciatica, and it does usually get better on its own. But this may actually make it more amenable to a placebo effect.

We know that the experience of pain is highly susceptible to expectation effects. Research shows that there is a very specific placebo analgesic process that occurs in specific brain pathways that reduce the activity in pain processing regions of the brain (Vase & Wartolowska, 2019). In one meta-analysis, it was shown that lower back pain, of the type that was probably experienced by Emily, shows pretty significant placebo effects (van Lennep et al., 2021). People suffering from pain, especially if it is intense, are more likely to place hope and expectations on anything they think may lead them to a bit of relief. From these high pain relief expectations, there can be an increase in the release of endogenous opioids in the body – such as endorphins – which are known to cause "feel good" sensations as well as pain relief (Vase & Wartolowska, 2019).

What Was the Actual Placebo?

Is the placebo just a tiny white pill, or is it a sham neurosurgery?[1] Research shows that the more invasive a placebo is, the larger it is, the more expensive it is – the more it works (Meissner & Linde, 2018). I would say that the price of finding someone to kidnap and kill, without getting caught, and then preparing the "substance" – makes human flesh a pretty expensive and invasive placebo. The fact that they are not just taking small pills, but eating the whole liver, licking brain sorbets, and rubbing themselves with human fat cream makes for a pretty impactful placebo experience.

> "IT'S CALLED THE PLACEBO EFFECT, you half brain-dead idi" – Holly Gibney
>
> (King, 2023, p.396)

⚠ **[Spoiler Alert]** And thus begins the final showdown between Holly and Rodney, as she shouts about placebo effects, and he shouts about their non-existence. It is almost a final countdown between the biomedical and biopsychosocial model. I will let you read the rest of the book to find out who wins – but you know who my money is on!

You Better Believe – *It*

For any constant reader, the mention of placebo effects should have immediately brought to mind *It* (see Box 4.2 for summary), and in particular, Eddie Kasparak and his all-powerful inhaler (referred to in the book as his aspirator). *It* must be mentioned in this chapter, as I hold that it was the placebo effect – or the idea of believing – that ultimately ⚠ **[Spoiler Alert]** defeated Pennywise (aka, It).

Box 4.2 *It*

It was my first experience with Stephen King material. Yes, the first time I read a Stephen King novel was *The Shining* in grad school, but it wasn't my first brush with King horror. That came in 1990, when I was 12, and

I watched the *It* miniseries on TV.[2] For many of us, Tim Curry's Pennywise is imprinted onto our amygdala (the part of the brain responsible for fear processing).

Needless to say, reading the actual novel was a scary prospect, especially at 1,169 pages. But read it I did, and as with many Constant Readers, I fell in love with The Losers Club.

It was published in 1986, and it tells the story of seven children (affectionately known as The Losers Club of 1958), who must battle an evil force haunting Derry, Maine – both when they are children and later as adults. The story weaves both the childhood and adult stories together, so we know that the children survived the ordeal in the 1950s – we are not so sure who will survive the second battle as adults.

[Spoiler Alert] The story begins in Derry, Maine in 1957, where Bill Denbrough, an 11-year-old boy, is helping his younger brother Georgie make a paper boat that he can play with outside during a rainstorm. Bill himself is feeling a bit under the weather, so he opts not to go out and help Georgie with the ship's maiden voyage down the street gutter. This is a choice that will haunt Bill later on – as Georgie, out on his own, is enticed into the gutter by Pennywise the Dancing Clown, who plies him with balloons and carnival sounds and smells. Pennywise, who is the embodiment of an evil that has haunted Derry for hundreds, if not thousands of years, murders Georgie.

Georgie is not the only child to be murdered or go missing, and it is during the summer of strict curfews and anxiety that The Losers Club comes together. The club consists of:

Bill Denbrough – aka "Stuttering Bill" – despite his stutter, Bill becomes the de facto leader of the group, and along with his trusty and speedy bike "Silver," motivates them to find the killer of his brother and vanquish the evil from Derry forever (or at least until the 1980s).

Eddie Kaspbrak – the youngest and shortest of the group, Eddie is plagued by asthma and a host of other ailments. His father died when he was young, and he was raised by an overprotective mother who is not too fond of the amount of time her Eddie spends with the Losers.

Richie Tozier – aka "Trashmouth" – the (non-evil) clown of the group. He is loud and crude and enjoys using a host of voices and impersonations, especially at times when it is not appropriate. Hence the development of the term "Beep-beep Richie" – which the Losers use to tell him to be quiet.

Stanley Uris – the quiet one, Stan is the one who tries to think the most logically and scientifically about what is happening in Derry. Ultimately, his inability to accept what he deems unacceptable causes him to break.

Beverly Marsh – the sole girl in the group, she is loved by all, especially Ben Hanscom. Smart and resourceful, Beverly deals with her own evils outside of Pennywise, as she tries to remain resilient despite having an abusive father and later an abusive husband.

Ben Hanscom – extremely shy and intelligent, Ben is also overweight as a child, which causes him to be a magnet for the bullies of Derry. For some reason, Ben really knows a lot about building dams, which endears him to the Losers, and he quickly becomes an integral part of the gang.

Mike Hanlon[3] – a latecomer to the Losers, Mike is Black, which causes him, like Ben, to be a target for the local bullies. It is during an attack by said bullies that Mike happens upon the Losers, who heroically protect and defend him in the infamous Apocalyptic Rock fight.

Then, as mentioned, we also have the bullies – the leader Henry Bowers, Victor Criss, Belch Huggins, Patrick Hockstetter, and the rest. While the bullies are a constant threat to the seven, so is It – the ancient evil that often takes the shape of Pennywise. It comes to each of the Losers as a manifestation of their particular fears, be it blood, lepers, werewolves, mummies, or giant birds.

After viewing one of Mike Hanlon's scrapbooks of historical events of Derry and performing a sweat lodge-type ritual in their clubhouse, the group realizes that they must fight the evil – which leads them to the sewer by the Derry Standpipe. Using their own powers of belief and connection, along with the help of Maturin, "the turtle of enormous girth,"[4] who created the earth, the Losers defeat the evil – for now. They swear a blood oath that if the evil should reappear, they will gather again to defeat it. And of course, 30 years later, that is exactly what happens.

Eddie is presented by Stephen King as the stereotypical allergy and asthma-prone individual. Yet this was not seen as "stereotypical" by the biomedical practitioners of the first half of the 20th century – it was seen as the medical truth. We have already discussed in Chapter 2 that asthma was seen as one of Alexander's "Holy Seven" – that is, it was seen as a mostly psychosomatic disorder – stemming from the mind, not the body. With this view in mind, medical practitioners felt there was nothing they could do for these patients – as they were focused on the body. Thus, the conclusion was that asthma, and allergy, and other related ailments had to do with the person – and that it was part of their personality (sounds sort of like the humoral theory we talked about in Chapter 2).

For example, physicians at the Tavistock Clinic in London proposed that there was an "allergic personality" in a 1938 paper. This person is generally a white male, who is upper-class and privileged, and who is apt to be of a "nervous temperament" (p.353). They are usually an only child, and their families are smaller in size. Children with this ailment have physical make-ups referred to as "delicate" (p.357). This is almost exactly the way that King describes Eddie.

There is also the issue of Eddie's overprotective and overbearing mother, Sonia. At the time, parents, and particularly mothers, were seen as problematic elements when it came to treating patients with asthma. In Chapter 1, we discussed parentectomies, where children were removed from their parents for long periods of time in hopes of improving their conditions. Franz Alexander himself insinuates that when someone with asthma wheezes – the wheeze is a cry out from having to deal with an overinvolved mother (Jackson, 2009). No wonder Eddie was wheezing so much!

If these were the accepted thoughts of the medical community at the time, it is no wonder that both Eddie's doctor and the pharmacists opted to assuage the over-involved mother and the delicate son by prescribing a HydrOx Mist – a placebo aspirator that consisted of hydrogen and oxygen (water) and a bit of camphor for that fresh medicinal smell. That smell is important, as we discussed in *Holly* – the more it looks and smells like medicine, the more likely it is to work.

Eddie's interaction with his mom, the doctor and the pharmacist, reminds me of a famous story that is often discussed in health psychology regarding the very earliest days of mind – body medicine. Ibn Sina (known in the West as Avicenna) was a philosopher physician who lived in central Asia in the late first century/early second century AD, and he is considered one of the fathers of medicine. Ibn Sina was very attuned to the mind – body connection, and he would use psychology to help him treat his patients (Hajar, 2013).

One of his most famous patients was a Persian prince who suffered from depression, became malnourished, and then began hallucinating he was a cow. As a cow, he refused to eat his family's food, insisting that they take him for slaughter so that they could be fed themselves. Ibn Sina was sent to treat the prince, and in an elaborate farce, he pretended to be a butcher about to kill the cow. At the last minute, Ibn Sina stopped, complaining that the cow was too skinny to be good for slaughter – and that it needed to fatten up to be useful. The story goes that the prince then began to eat and gain strength and weight – and when he got to a healthy enough condition, he stopped believing he was a cow and was cured.

As stated, at the time Eddie Kasparak and his mother are living in Derry, asthma was considered to be mostly "in the head" – just like the Persian prince's cow delusion. In essence, what Eddie's doctor and pharmacists are doing – by offering him a "medicine" that is just water and some camphor – is pretending to be a butcher. The pharmacist and the doctor have been playing a bit of Ibn Sina, thinking it will protect both Eddie and his mother from the truth about his "mental weakness." When it looks like the deception isn't helping Eddie anymore, the pharmacist decides to come clean and tell him that the aspirator has been a placebo all this time. This does not help.

However, here is where I think the doctor and pharmacist got it wrong. Their assumption is that there is nothing physically wrong with Eddie, and the fact that the placebo they prescribed helps him further proves their point. I disagree. Eddie could very well have asthma, and the placebo could be working – they don't discount each other. In one study, Kemeny and colleagues (2007) looked at participants who had been clinically diagnosed as having mild intermittent or persistent asthma. All participants, over the course of six weeks, received either an inhaler containing Salmeterol (a bronchodilator) for three weeks, or an inhaler with the Salmeterol removed for three weeks. They were randomized to which weeks they would receive which condition (first three weeks or second) – so all were exposed to both the medication and the placebo, just at different times – we call this a crossover design.

At the end of each of the three weeks, the participants underwent a methacholine challenge – they were exposed to methacholine to induce an asthma attack like airway narrowing. They then looked at whether being on the Salmeterol for three weeks or placebo for three weeks prevented the narrowing due to the exposure. What they found was that 18% of the participants were highly responsive to the placebo; that is, taking the placebo itself was able to prevent the reduction in airway flow that was expected to occur in response to the methacholine. That is pretty amazing – the placebo basically prevented them from having an asthma attack!

The fact that people with asthma can benefit from placebos has been repeatedly shown (Dutile et al., 2014; Luc, 2019). Many factors could lead to this result. We know that placebos cause the release of endorphins, and some research has shown that endorphins could potentially mediate chronic asthma symptoms (in mice at least, see Pandey et al., 2023). However, I think there is something even more relevant to consider, and it is something I have thought about a lot in my own research. When you really think about it – what is the one system that we truly have control over as humans? I can't say to you – "hey – stop your endocrine system from working, now!" or "you better put that reproductive system on hold" – trust me, my premenopausal self wishes we had such control over those systems! The only time this ever works is when we say "hold your breath." And we can do this. We can consciously stop breathing for a period of time. For me, the respiratory system is tied to our mind in more complex ways than science has yet to explain, but this control is telling. If I can tell my lungs to stop taking in air, then my expectation that a placebo can help those lungs take in more air just makes sense to me. If my mind believes that there is more air and that I can breathe better, then the communication between lungs and brain is going to make this more apt to happen.

And this brings me to my last point about placebos – they are good! I don't think of them as some kind of "effect" that is an afterthought in a biomedical model, or just a means to an end in a biopsychosocial one. A placebo is something that we can really use to make our lives better. As long as it doesn't harm you or someone else (like say, cannibalism) or it is illegal (like say, cannibalism), we should be using it as much as possible, as it can make our lives better, in whatever way it works. For instance, as I am writing this, I am drinking a smoothie, and I had the smoothie maker boost it with the "Brain Smart Booster." Now, there is no way that I think, with my evidence-based mind, that whatever that booster contains is going to actually make me think better. But it has just put a little bit of expectancy in my mind, and now I am pumping out this paragraph like it was nothing! And yes, research shows that the placebo effect can work – even when you know it is a placebo (Schaefer et al., 2018).

Sometimes, when I am working with my clients, they might dismiss when they are feeling better with "it is probably just the placebo effect." First of all, "just" the placebo effect? No, it is a complicated mind – body interaction that deserves our respect. Second – who cares? The placebo effect is just as legitimate of a reason for feeling better than any other. My boy Eddie understood this. It doesn't matter that the aspirator only contained water and camphor – it helped him. ⚠ **[Spoiler Alert]** And when he needed that aspirator to contain battery acid to fight off a giant eye – it did – saving them all.

Voodoo Death and Nocebo Effects – *Thinner*

Now, let me step off of my placebo soapbox to introduce the darker side of the placebo story – the nocebo. While placebos deal with positive expectations leading to positive outcomes, nocebos are about our negative expectations leading to negative outcomes (Colloca, 2024). While the term nocebo was first used by a doctor named Walter Kennedy in 1961, I think we need to start with another Walter, one we talked about in previous chapters – Walter Cannon.

Voodoo Death

If you remember, Walter Cannon was the Harvard doctor who coined the term "fight or flight" – he was instrumental in our understanding of how emotions impact us physiologically. In 1942, he published an article in *American Anthropologist* where he describes "Voodoo Death." The article discusses (in a way not too politically correct these days) how certain populations of people across the globe believe in curses, magic, sorcery, hexes, etc., and then they actually die from those things. Cannon cites anthropological findings of medicine men condemning men to death, and then those men die via supernatural means. Medical doctors who have witnessed these phenomena claim that those who have died by these magical means have probably died from fear. Cannon asks – can fear kill someone? Is this how someone dies a "voodoo death?"

There are many ways that one can be affected when a curse has been placed on them, a curse that they fully believe in, based on their culture and upbringing. First, of course, is the feeling of fear one has because of the assumption that death is imminent. Cannon states that a natural reaction to that fear would be a lack of appetite – the afflicted person may refuse to eat or drink – weakening their body. Along with these behavioral factors, there can also be extreme changes to the body's stress systems – specifically the HPA and SAM axis. The idea that Cannon had was that the fear experienced by those who were cursed was so extreme – it induced sympathetic activation so severe that the person would go into "shock." That shock was similar to what was experienced by those wounded in World War I. This shock would lead to profound constriction of blood vessels, reducing blood flow and blood pressure,[5] that when coupled with the weakened body, caused the death of the individual.

When that person died from the fear – the people around them believed that they had died from the curse, making everyone even more likely to believe in the power of the curse (this would be learning by association). This reinforcement made people even more afraid when a curse was placed on them, and thus more likely to die from it. Thus, we have an early explanation of the mechanism of the nocebo effect – that with negative expectations come biopsychosocial changes that then lead to negative outcomes.

Not mentioned yet are the social mechanisms underlying this. Biologically, we have fear instigating changes in HPA and SAM axes, among others. Psychologically, we have the person emotionally distraught – to the point of not eating or drinking. Another common occurrence here is the social impact – people who experience such curses will often see rejection by their community. They are ostracized due to whatever "evil" thing they did to make a curse necessary, or because people are choosing to "protect" themselves. Therefore, there is no one there to take care of them, make sure they eat, provide social support and comfort, and so forth, increasing the likelihood that the curse will be fatal.

Now that we have a better understanding of the historical underpinnings of nocebo effects, let's get into more details by exploring the horrifying curse that befalls Bill Halleck in Stephen King's *Thinner* (see Box 4.3 for summary).

Box 4.3 *Thinner*

In 1984, *Thinner* was published under King's alter ego, Richard Bachman (see details in Chapter 3). It is the story of William "Billy" Halleck – a rather obese lawyer who is the husband of Heidi and father to teenaged Linda (who has a pretty bad case of acne, see Box 4.4). The family lives in the affluent town of Fairview, Connecticut, and when a nomadic group of Romani people[6] come into town, the locals are not thrilled. However, this does not upset the Hallecks too much, until one fateful night when Billy and Heidi are distractedly driving through town, and hit an elderly Romani woman.

⚠ **[Spoiler Alert]** The woman dies from her injuries, and due to his status and connections within the community, Billy is not held accountable. This angers Taduz Lemke, the father (yes, father!) of the elderly woman. As Billy is leaving the courthouse on the day his manslaughter charge is dismissed, he is approached by Taduz, who simply whispers the word "thinner" as he gently touches Billy's cheek. This curse is what will wreak havoc on Billy throughout the rest of the novel.

Billy was in desperate need of shaving off a few pounds anyway, and at first, his weight loss was a welcome occurrence, which nobody seemed to question. Yet when the weight loss continues, and even speeds up, Billy finds himself worried – is it cancer? After many medical tests, the answer is no – not cancer. Billy is haunted by the one word whispered by the grieving Romani father, "thinner," and begins to suspect that the man may have put some kind of curse on him.

Billy finds out that several of the people involved in his sham of a court hearing have also had their own medical emergencies – the police officer who covered for him has a crippling case of acne, and the judge develops a grotesque skin condition. Billy discovers that they were both approached by

Taduz after the court hearing, just like he was. After both men take their own lives, Billy decides it is time to act.

Billy reaches out to a friend and former client – Richie Grinnelli. Richie, also known as "The Hammer," is heavily involved in organized crime, and has a wealth of resources at his disposal. He is able to find the current location of the nomadic Lemke family, who have long left Billy and Fairview behind. Billy uses this info to track them down and tries to get Taduz to lift the thinner curse – without success. He even takes a ball-bearing through his hand for his trouble. Billy is now not just severely emaciated but he is also significantly wounded.

Understanding his dire condition, Billy calls in reinforcements, and Richie arrives with much enthusiasm to help. Richie then embarks on a manic campaign of harassment against the Lemkes, until they agree to remove the curse. Since the curse cannot be removed outright, it must be transferred into another object – in this case a strawberry pie. Whoever eats the strawberry pie will then be cursed "thinner." For what happens after this, it is up to the intrepid reader (or Googler) to find out.

Expect Thinner, Be Thinner

I believe Walter Cannon would say that Billy fell victim to a voodoo curse. We could also say that the whisper of the word "thinner" acted as a nocebo. Nocebo effects are common in clinical trials when the potential side effects of a medication are mentioned. You are told that the experimental medication may cause headaches, fatigue, and dry mouth. You are then randomly assigned to the control condition (you receive a sugar pill instead of the medication), and while taking it, you experience headaches, fatigue, and dry mouth. This is a classic nocebo effect.

Just like a placebo effect, there are many factors that are likely to make a nocebo effect more likely to happen. Colloca (2024) presents multiple external (negative verbal suggestions, social observations, and contextual factors) and internal factors that play a role in the presence and size of a nocebo effect. Let's go through a few of them and see how they apply to Billy Halleck.

Negative Verbal Suggestions – this one is pretty obvious. On the most basic level, what Taduz Lemke did was whisper a side effect to Billy. It takes a while for this to sink in, but once it does, it is hard for Billy to let it go.

Social Observation – this is when you see other people experiencing a negative side effect; you are more likely to experience it as well. Billy really started to believe in his weight loss side effect when he saw what befell Duncan Hopley (the police chief) and Cary Rossington (the judge). ⚠ **[Spoiler Alert]** Seeing that they had been cursed, and the severity of their "side effects," really amped up Billy's fear and expectations. When both of the men died, we return to that associative learning I talked about with Cannon – now he has associated curses with death, and his fight or flight response may be in overdrive, making his weight loss more impactful.

Contextual factors – context matters, and if it was just some random person on the street who whispered "thinner," we wouldn't have a horror novel to talk about. Taduz Lemke is an old man – I mean really old, well into his 100s. This is the first set of context Billy has to go by. This guy is old, he has seen some things and been through some things. You can also guess that he is pretty angry about the death of his daughter, and the fact that no one in the town really cared. He has motivation, and motivation that Billy is fully aware of. He also has a horrifying rotting nose, which really makes him, and what he represents for Billy, quite salient. One last contextual factor that really imparted to Billy the efficacy of the curse – Taduz Lemke and his family are from a group of people stereotypically seen as people who believe in curses. If they believe in it so fully, it is hard to see how that belief would not rub off on those around them.

Internal factors – what is it about Billy that makes him more susceptible to the nocebo effects of the curse? First off, Billy is male and may be more prone to the verbal suggestions that impact nocebo expectations (Colloca, 2024). I also believe he is suffering from some negative affect after getting away with vehicular manslaughter. I think he is feeling guilty for the death, as well as guilty for getting away with it. He is also having some pretty intense feelings of anger over his wife and the role she played in the accident. We know that these negative moods and appraisals can make negative expectations more likely to manifest.

In essence, it is a perfect storm of external and internal factors that lead to the biological fear response, the psychological expectations, and ultimately the social isolation (Billy eventually winds up alone in a hotel, hundreds of miles away from his family) that comes with the nocebo curse. Now, the question is – will the eater of the strawberry pie have the same experience?

Box 4.4 Linda Halleck's Complexion

Within the first few pages of *Thinner*, we are introduced to Linda Halleck, the teenage daughter of Billy. After her father hits and kills the old women, Linda experiences some bullying at school. Billy notices that during this stressful time, she doesn't eat, and "her complexion had flared up" (King, 2016, p. 4). The idea that being under extreme stress can cause acne flare-ups has been around a long time, but is it true? One thing that has been found repeatedly in the research is that the presence of acne is associated with poor psychological outcomes. In one systematic review and meta-analysis, it was shown that among 42 studies, acne was significantly associated with both depression and anxiety (Samuels et al., 2020). It can be particularly detrimental to self-esteem, especially among women (Gallitano & Berson, 2018).

But what about psychological stress causing acne? Many people report that it does, and studies that use self-reported stress and self-reported acne breakouts bear this out (Jović et al., 2017). It seems that there are multiple potential biological pathways by which stress can get "under the skin" and cause skin problems (Passeron et al., 2021). One such pathway could be the HPA axis, which we discussed in Chapter 1. The influx of hormones from the system can upset skin balance, particularly glucocorticoids (cortisol), increasing the production of sebum. Sebum is a substance produced by the glands in your skin (known as the sebaceous glands). It is meant to protect and moisturize, but too much of it can result in acne.

In one interesting study, researchers followed university students throughout an academic quarter to see if their acne was reactive to exam stress (Chiu et al., 2003). Using digital photographs of their skin, each student's acne was rated for severity based on a common dermatological technique. The study found that those students who reported the highest increases in stress during their exam periods showed the highest increase in their acne severity. These results controlled for sleeping and eating habits, which is a good indicator that stress itself was causing the acne changes, not the behaviors that resulted from the stress.

What does all this mean? Chances are Linda was having an acne flare-up due to the stress caused by the bullying. Luckily for Linda, this particular stressor did not last long. Little does she know, however, what is in store for her as the curse starts digging its claws into her father. I am sure her face probably will not appreciate the curse any more than Billy Halleck does.

I hope that this chapter has convinced you of the power of placebo and nocebo effects, and how they act as a great example of mind – body interactions. And just so you know, research shows that if you rip out this page and eat it, your (insert ailment here) will be cured. Try it out and let me know how it goes! (Just kidding, please don't do that).

Versions of *Holly*

Novel: King, S. (2023). *Holly*. Scribner.
Audiobook: King, S. (2023). *Holly* [Audiobook]. Simon & Schuster Audio. (Narrator, J., Lupe).

Versions of *It*

Novel: King, S. (1986). *It*. Viking Press.
Miniseries: Wallace, T. L. Director). (1990). *It* [TV miniseries]. Warner Bros. Television.
Films:
Muschietti, A. (Director). (2017). *It* [Film]. Warner Bros. Pictures.
Muschietti, A. (Director). (2019). *It Chapter Two* [Film]. Warner Bros. Pictures.
Audiobook: King, S. (1986). *It* [Audiobook]. Simon & Schuster Audio. (Narrator, S., Weber).

Versions of *Thinner*[7]

Novel: Bachman, R. (1984). *Thinner*. NAL Books.
Film: Holland, T. (Director). (1996). *Thinner* [Film]. Paramount Pictures.[8]
Audiobook: Bachman, R. (1984). *Thinner* [Audiobook]. Simon & Schuster Audio. (Narrator, F., Muller).

Further Exploration Questions

1 When reading *Holly*, what other factors do you see that make the human flesh placebo such a strong one for Emily and Rodney Harris? Research has also found that certain personalities are more likely to have placebo responses than others (see Kern et al., 2020) – do they fit any of the "placebo-prone" personality traits?
2 What other characters in Stephen King's work meet the criteria for an "allergic personality"? What about in other works of fiction, or TV shows and movies? Do you think this is a fair categorization? Why or why not?

Notes

1 Yes, sham neurosurgeries are performed. If you want to know whether your neurosurgical procedure (like electromagnetic stimulation) actually works, you need to compare it to as similar a placebo as possible. So instead of taking a real pill and a sugar pill – you get a neurosurgery with some stimulation, or a neurosurgery without (the sham; see Bond et al., 2016, for an example).
2 This is one of those events that we have in life that we will always blame our parents for. How could my mom let me watch this? I also blame my mom for letting me watch the Richard Harris movie *Orca* when I was even younger. Now I have an unreasonable fear of both Eldritch clowns and killer whales. Thanks mom!
3 We will meet Mike Hanlon again in Chapter 9 – as the head librarian in Derry, he is one of the "weak" social ties that provide Ralph Roberts with information support for his insomnia.
4 This all sounds a bit trippy, I know. This description of Maturin comes from *The Dark Tower* Series. But Maturin is an important character within the Stephen King macroverse, and Maturin is an eternal enemy of It, so I needed to mention the turtle to appease the Beam.
5 You might remember from the first chapter that when stress activates hormone release through the HPA and SAM axes, we see INCREASES in blood pressure. This is the part that Cannon got incorrectly (as we understand it today).
6 We will use this term in place of the more outdated and offensive term used throughout the novel.
7 Since King published *Thinner* under his pseudonym Richard Bachman, I have used that citation here. However, if you are looking for the book or audiobook, you can find many editions using the name Stephen King as the author.
8 I am not sure what to say about the movie version of *Thinner*, except to watch it if you would like a laugh (not a scare).

Bibliography

Bond, A. E., Dallapiazza, R., Huss, D., Warren, A. L., Sperling, S., Gwinn, R., … & Elias, W. J. (2016). 132 A randomized, sham-controlled trial of transcranial magnetic resonance-guided focused ultrasound thalamotomy trial for the treatment of tremor-dominant, idiopathic Parkinson disease. *Neurosurgery*, *63*, 154. https://doi.org/10.1227/01.neu.0000489702.18785.5f

Cannon, W. B. (1942). "Voodoo" death. *American Anthropologist*, *44*(2), 169–181. https://www.jstor.org/stable/663018 https://doi.org/10.1525/aa.1942.44.2.02a00010

Chiu, A., Chon, S. Y., & Kimball, A. B. (2003). The response of skin disease to stress: Changes in the severity of acne vulgaris as affected by examination stress. *Archives of Dermatology*, *139*(7), 897–900. https://doi.org/10.1001/archderm.139.7.897

Colloca, L. (2024). The nocebo effect. *Annual Review of Pharmacology and Toxicology*, *64*(1), 171–190. https://doi.org/10.1146/annurev-pharmtox-022723-112425

Colloca, L., & Miller, F. G. (2011). How placebo responses are formed: A learning perspective. *Philosophical Transactions of the Royal Society B: Biological Sciences*, *366*(1572), 1859–1869. https://doi.org/10.1098/rstb.2010.0398

Dutile, S., Kaptchuk, T. J., & Wechsler, M. E. (2014). The placebo effect in asthma. *Current Allergy and Asthma Reports*, *14*(8), 456. https://doi.org/10.1007/s11882-014-0456-2

Gallitano, S. M., & Berson, D. S. (2018). How acne bumps cause the blues: The influence of acne vulgaris on self-esteem. *International Journal of Women's Dermatology*, *4*(1), 12–17. https://doi.org/10.1016/j.ijwd.2017.10.004

Hafliðadóttir, S. H., Juhl, C. B., Nielsen, S. M., Henriksen, M., Harris, I. A., Bliddal, H., & Christensen, R. (2021). Placebo response and effect in randomized clinical trials: Meta-research with focus on contextual effects. *Trials*, *22*(1), 493. https://doi.org/10.1186/s13063-021-05454-8

Hajar R., & M. D. (2013). The air of history (part v) Ibn Sina (Avicenna): The great physician and philosopher. *Heart Views: The Official Journal of the Gulf Heart Association*, *14*(4), 196–201. https://doi.org/10.4103/1995-705X.126893

Howe, L. C., Goyer, J. P., & Crum, A. J. (2017). Harnessing the placebo effect: Exploring the influence of physician characteristics on placebo response. *Health Psychology*, *36*(11), 1074. https://doi.org/10.1037/hea0000499

Jackson, M. (2009). *Asthma: The biography*. Oxford University Press.

Jović, A., Marinović, B., Kostović, K., Čeović, R., Basta-Juzbašić, A., & Bukvić Mokos, Z. (2017). The impact of psychological stress on acne. *Acta Dermatovenerologica Croatica*, *25*(2), 133–133. PMID: 28871928

Kemeny, M. E., Rosenwasser, L. J., Panettieri, R. A., Rose, R. M., Berg-Smith, S. M., & Kline, J. N. (2007). Placebo response in asthma: A robust and objective phenomenon. *Journal of Allergy and Clinical Immunology*, *119*(6), 1375–1381. https://doi.org/10.1016/j.jaci.2007.03.016

Kennedy, W. P. (1961). The nocebo reaction. *Medical World*, *95*, 203–205.

Kern, A., Kramm, C., Witt, C. M., & Barth, J. (2020). The influence of personality traits on the placebo/nocebo response: A systematic review. *Journal of Psychosomatic Research*, *128*, 109866. https://doi.org/10.1016/j.jpsychores.2019.109866

King, S. (2016). *Thinner*. Scribner. https://www.amazon.com/dp/B01M0JYJ7D

King, S. (2023). *Holly*. Scribner. https://www.amazon.com/dp/B0BHTZ8J9F

Luc, F., Prieur, E., Whitmore, G. A., Gibson, P. G., Vandemheen, K. L., & Aaron, S. D. (2019). Placebo effects in clinical trials evaluating patients with uncontrolled persistent asthma. *Annals of the American Thoracic Society*, *16*(9), 1124–1130. https://doi.org/10.1513/AnnalsATS.201901-071OC

Meissner, K., & Linde, K. (2018). Are blue pills better than green? How treatment features modulate placebo effects. *International Review of Neurobiology*, *139*, 357–378. https://doi.org/10.1016/bs.irn.2018.07.014

Pandey, V., Yadav, V., Singh, R., Srivastava, A., & Subhashini. (2023). β-Endorphin (an endogenous opioid) inhibits inflammation, oxidative stress and apoptosis via Nrf-2 in asthmatic murine model. *Scientific Reports*, *13*(1), 12414. https://doi.org/10.1038/s41598-023-38366-5

Passeron, T., Zouboulis, C. C., Tan, J., Andersen, M. L., Katta, R., Lyu, X., … & Peters, E. M. J. (2021). Adult skin acute stress responses to short-term environmental and internal aggression from exposome factors. *Journal of the European Academy of Dermatology and Venereology*, *35*(10), 1963–1975. https://doi.org/10.1111/jdv.17432

Samuels, D. V., Rosenthal, R., Lin, R., Chaudhari, S., & Natsuaki, M. N. (2020). Acne vulgaris and risk of depression and anxiety: A meta-analytic review. *Journal of the American Academy of Dermatology*, *83*(2), 532–541. https://doi.org/10.1016/j.jaad.2020.02.040

Schaefer, M., Sahin, T., & Berstecher, B. (2018). Why do open-label placebos work? A randomized controlled trial of an open-label placebo induction with and without extended information about the placebo effect in allergic rhinitis. *PloS One*, *13*(3), e0192758. https://doi.org/10.1371/journal.pone.0192758

Valat, J. P., Genevay, S., Marty, M., Rozenberg, S., & Koes, B. (2010). Sciatica. *Best Practice & Research Clinical Rheumatology*, *24*(2), 241–252. https://doi.org/10.1016/j.berh.2009.11.005

van Lennep, J. H. P. A., Trossèl, F., Perez, R. S. G. M., Otten, R. H. J., van Middendorp, H., Evers, A. W. M., & Szadek, K. M. (2021). Placebo effects in low back pain: A systematic review and meta-analysis of the literature. *European Journal of Pain*, *25*(9), 1876–1897. https://doi.org/10.1002/ejp.1811

Vase, L., & Wartolowska, K. (2019). Pain, placebo, and test of treatment efficacy: A narrative review. *British Journal of Anaesthesia*, *123*(2), e254–e262. https://doi.org/10.1016/j.bja.2019.01.040

Wittkower, E., & Berlin, M. D. (1938). Studies in hay-fever patients (the allergic personality). *Journal of Mental Science*, *84*(349), 352–369. https://doi.org/10.1192/bjp.84.349.352

5 Character Development

The Health Psychology of Bill Hodges

Bill Hodges, Det.-Ret

When we first meet Bill Hodges in the novel *Mr. Mercedes* (see Box 5.1 for a summary of the trilogy), things are not going so well for him. He is sitting on his Lay Z Boy lounger, watching some daytime TV, his gun sitting next to him on the side table. The title of this introductory chapter is called Det.-Ret. – meaning detective, retired. We can see how this new identity has taken a toll on Bill Hodges. This new label tells us a lot about his potential mindset and his potential health.

> **Box 5.1 The Bill Hodges Trilogy**
>
> The Bill Hodges Trilogy is a set of novels that revolve around Kermit William Hodges, known as Bill, a retired police detective in an unidentified Ohio city. Bill is a divorced, white male, in his late 60s, when we first meet him.
>
> **Book 1: *Mr. Mercedes* (2014)**
>
> The *Mr. Mercedes* of the title refers to one of the last cases Bill Hodges had when he was a police detective – and one that was still unsolved when he retired. Mr. Mercedes was the name given to the driver of a Mercedes that plowed into a crowd of early-morning job seekers at a city-sponsored job fair. Many people are killed and maimed, and the driver in the hit-and-run has never been identified. Bill eventually retires, haunted by the fact that Mr. Mercedes is the one that got away on his watch.
>
> However, about six months into his retirement, he receives a letter from Mr. Mercedes, commenting on Bill's absence from the case. He also teases Bill with the fact that one of his first suspects, Olivia Trelawney, who owned the Mercedes, has taken her own life. Bill's zest for the chase is renewed by this letter, and instead of going to the police with it, he begins his own private investigation.
>
> Through this investigation, he meets Olivia's sister Janey and Janey's cousin Holly. Along with Bill's neighbor, Jerome Robinson, they all become

DOI: 10.4324/9781003495994-5

intricately involved in Bill's investigation. This investigation eventually leads to Brady Hartsfield, a young man who has been driving the popular ice cream truck through Bill's neighborhood (keeping an eye on him), as well as working at the local big box electronics store.

⚠ **[Spoiler Alert]** The letter that Brady wrote to Bill was meant to discourage him, and Brady had hoped that Bill would take his own life – and is surprised that it did the opposite. Brady ups his game and continues to taunt Bill through a website called "Debbie's Blue Umbrella." In addition, he successfully blows up Bill's car when Janey is in it and attempts an unsuccessful poisoning of Jerome's dog. His failure to kill Bill with the car bomb, and his accidental poisoning of his mother with the dog poison, leads Brady to become suicidal himself. However, his suicide plans include collateral damage, and he prepares to blow himself up at a boy band concert.

Luckily for the pre-teens attending the concert – Bill, Jerome, and Holly end up discovering his plans and foil his plot just before detonation. Holly is the one who successfully beats Brady into a coma using a sock filled with ball-bearings (what Bill refers to as a Happy Slapper) she had been carrying with her. This last-minute save provides praise for Holly and Jerome, and Bill is not punished for his extracurricular police activities.

Book 2: *Finders Keepers* (2015)

Finders Keepers refers to the private investigation firm that is started by Bill Hodges after the events of *Mr. Mercedes*. Holly joins the agency, and Jerome works with them both on occasion. Bill, Holly, and Jerome become entwined with a teenage boy named Pete Saubers – whose father was injured in the Mr. Mercedes massacre. Pete has found a trunk filled with notebooks and a lot of money, which his family could desperately use due to the injuries sustained by his father. Peter deftly provides the money to his family without them being any the wiser, and he becomes obsessed with the notebooks he found with the money.

After reading through the notebooks, Pete begins to understand that these are the writings of John Rothstein, a famous writer who was brutally murdered decades ago, and whose killer was never caught. We learn that Rothstein was killed by a rather unstable fan, who stole the money, as well as all of the notebooks, and buried them in the trunk for safekeeping. Unfortunately, this fan, Morris Bellamy, is shortly arrested for other crimes, and does not get the chance to read his favorite (or is it most detested?) author's notebooks. He spends decades in jail dreaming about the trunk, and the written treasures it holds.

⚠ **[Spoiler Alert]** Eventually, Morris is released from prison and begins his search for his trunk. He then finds out that someone has found the trunk and taken it for themselves. At the same time, Bill, Holly, and Jerome are investigating what is going on with Pete Saubers at the behest of his sister. Everything comes to a head when Morris finds out that Pete is the one who spent his money and read his favorite (detested?) author's notebooks. Morris sets off to find Pete and make him pay.

Lucky for Pete, Bill, Holly, and Jerome are good at their work, and they figure out what has been going on just in time. A final confrontation leads to another criminal's death, and Finders Keepers with another win.

Book 3: *End of Watch* (2016)

While the Pete Saubers/Morris Bellamy case was going on, Brady Hartsfield remained in a coma in a special clinic for brain injuries. Bill has been going to visit him on a regular basis, much to everyone's disapproval. Brady eventually becomes aware of these visits from Bill, as a new experimental drug has him slowly waking up – and being possessed of extrasensory powers – his mind can control and move things around him – including other people.

⚠ **[Spoiler Alert]** At the same time, survivors of the Mr. Mercedes killings start to take their own lives, and Finders Keepers is on the case. They discover that a discontinued handheld gaming computer called the "Zappit" has been at the scenes of all of the suicides, including the attempted suicide of Jerome's sister Barbara. Holly eventually learns that Brady is at the center of the Zappits and their power over vulnerable people and is able to end his psychic attacks – as well as him – for good.

The Presenting Problem

When it comes to the health psychology of Bill Hodges, it is difficult to know where to start. So let's start where a health care provider would begin – at the presenting problem. The presenting problem is what we call the initial complaint, the reason the person is seeking help. Of course, Bill is not seeking help, but if we were assessing him based on how he is feeling when we first meet him, I would say that the presenting problem is depression and accompanying suicidality. We aren't the only ones picking up on this – it seems that Brady Hartsfield, the Mercedes killer, has also picked up on this from simply watching Bill Hodges outside his house.

What are the signs and symptoms that Bill is exhibiting? Signs are objective observations we can make concerning what is going on, while symptoms are what Bill subjectively experiences. Table 5.1 presents the signs and symptoms we can first pick up on when Bill is introduced to us, sitting in his easy chair, watching a Jerry Springer-esque TV program.

Table 5.1 Bill Hodges Presenting Problem Intake

Bill Hodges Initial Intake – Presenting Signs and Symptoms	
Signs – objective Observations made regarding Bill Hodges' current condition.	• Gun next to him on side table, touches gun. • Picks up gun, looks into the barrel, sometimes puts into his mouth. • Afternoon shows – has watched every day since his retirement (six months ago). • Sleep disruption – has been going to bed late. • Poor diet.
Symptoms – subjective Bill Hodges' own insight into what he is experiencing.	• Bill thinks about the suicide of the TV show host. • Has chosen a particular gun that "never jams" to be next to him, easily accessible, as opposed to his other gun. • Has lost interest in drinking alcohol. • Knows he puts a gun into his mouth to "get used to it." • Has the urge to commit suicide, thinks it might pass if he gives it time. • Can't sleep – reports of rumination. • Reports he does not enjoy the taste of the "meals" he makes.

As you can see, there are several objective observations we can make regarding what is going on with Bill Hodges, as well as his own subjective insight. These signs and symptoms indicate that, according to the American Psychiatric Association's Diagnostic and Statistical Manual of Mental Disorders (DSM-5, 2013),[1] Bill may be experiencing Major Depressive Disorder (MDD). In order for one to be diagnosed with MDD, several criteria have to be met. First, symptoms (we usually discuss symptoms here, as we usually use patient self-report as the basis of a diagnosis, at least for adults) must be present every day for at least two weeks. I think that Bill has this down, as his signs and symptoms have been present for six months since his retirement.

Next, the symptoms must include either a depressed mood or a loss of interest in things that the person once found pleasure in. While I am not sure we have enough data to make a conclusion about a depressed mood, Bill has definitely lost interest in things he once loved – such as eating and drinking. Throughout this book, we also see him returning to things that he had previously lost interest in, like singing some Bob Seger when the mood strikes.

The DSM-5 lists nine criteria, two of which are the required depressed mood or loss of interest mentioned above. The other seven are: changes to weight and/or appetite, sleep disruptions (either too much or too little), psychomotor changes observed by others, fatigue or loss of energy, feelings of guilt or worthlessness, difficulties thinking or concentrating, and recurrent thoughts of suicide and death. The diagnosis requires five or more of these nine criteria.

As already discussed, Bill meets the criteria of loss of interest. It is also pretty clear that he has been having recurrent thoughts of suicide, even going as far as keeping his gun as close to him as possible and sometimes placing it in his mouth. He has sleep difficulties, and one of the things that happens when he can't sleep is that he ruminates on the cases he didn't solve, the things he did wrong, and so forth (feelings of guilt and worthlessness). That takes care of two more criteria. We have strong evidence that he meets four of the five criteria, but it is unclear whether an official diagnosis could be made here. Regardless, it is clear that we can safely say that Bill Hodges is presenting with depressive-like symptoms and suicidality.

The Problem with Not Working

Shortly after we are given this introduction to Det-Ret Hodges, he receives the taunting letter from Brady, who is hoping to push Bill over the edge – teasing him into pulling the trigger on the.38 Smith & Wesson. What ends up happening is just the opposite, and it is through this miscalculation on Brady's part that we gain further insight into the causes of Bill's depression and suicidality.

Our first clue as to the etiology (aka cause) of Bill's condition is that it started six months ago, right after he fully retired from detective work. Research regarding retirement is mixed – some recent meta-analyses have shown retirement is associated with increased depression (Li et al., 2021), while others show that retirement actually protects people from depression (Odone et al., 2021). What might be more important for us to look at here is not retirement per se, but purpose in life.

Purpose in life is an important theoretical concept in health psychology. At its most basic level, it is defined as how much of the life currently experienced by the individual is guided and influenced by the person's values and life goals (Kim et al., 2019). In essence, purpose in life is about feeling that your life is moving in a meaningful direction. Using data from the Health and Retirement Study (people 50 and older), Kim and colleagues (2022) found that those who reported the highest levels of purpose in life had significantly reduced risk of death, stroke, lung disease, and cognitive impairment when compared to those with the lowest levels. High purpose in life was also associated with higher activity levels and reduced sleep problems. From this study, it seems that having a purpose in life is hugely important when it comes to one's health and well-being. Unfortunately for Bill, it seems that since retiring from the police force, he has a life that does not seem to be guided by any values and goals, let alone ones he finds meaningful.

One study that seems pertinent to Bill's condition was conducted by Bonnewyn and colleagues (2014) on a set of older patients Belgium. They asked these patients questions about their life attitudes, including purpose in life. They used a seven-point Likert scale, which asks people if they agree with a statement on a scale from one, meaning strongly agree, to seven, meaning strongly disagree. The questions came from the Life Attitude Profile – Revised (LAP-R; Reker, 1992) and included "In thinking about my life, I see a reason for my being here" or "My past achievements have given my life purpose and meaning." It is clear that when we first meet Bill, he would probably answer with a 1 – strongly disagree. The researchers then assessed the patient's wish to die. They divided the participants between those who had a death wish and those who did not, and they found that those with a death wish scored significantly lower on purpose in life. This relationship was stronger for males than for females.

This leads me to believe that it wasn't retirement itself that was impacting Bill, but the loss of purpose that resulted when he stopped working. Unwittingly, Brady's taunting letter brings Bill back to himself and his goals, and with it, we see him letting go of the death wish that had been haunting him.

The Problems with Working

Yes, as we have seen, there are problems with Bill not working. But there are also problems that arise from his working, and the type of work he used to do, and is currently pursuing in his retirement. As previously stated, Bill Hodges has spent the majority of his life in law enforcement – approximately 40 years, 27 of those years as a detective. This is a particularly long time, as even Bill himself recognizes. Most of the law enforcement officers (LEOs) he has worked with retire after 25 or 30 years. Even before he was a police officer himself, he lived with the lifestyle, as his father was a "beat cop."[2]

This is a long time to be involved in police work. According to the U.S. Department of Labor, "police and detective work can be physically demanding, stressful, and dangerous" (Bureau of Labor Statistics, 2025). A lot of policework involves vigilance – being in a state of high alert – sustaining your attention for a period of time so that you are more responsive to the stimuli around you (Klösch et al., 2022). Vigilance is mentally and physically taxing, and it may be one of the reasons that police officers have higher mortality rates from cardiovascular disease (CVD), cirrhosis of the liver, and mental disorders (Violanti et al., 2021).

The liver cirrhosis statistic is relevant to Bill, as he has stated that when he was on the force, "he was damned near an alcoholic" (King, 2014, p.19). The abuse of alcohol by LEOs was shown to be associated with work-related traumatic distress, and an avoidance of that distress (Chopko et al., 2013). While he may not admit it, I believe Bill has experienced work-related distress, and he has listed out within this book the kind of things he has been exposed to on the job: bum fighting, killers, robbery gangs, arsonists, rapists, and so forth. Most obviously, he is haunted by the Mr. Mercedes case, which involved a horrifying crime scene that included multiple mutilated bodies, including a baby.

The drinking and the job also ruined Bill's relationship with his now ex-wife and daughter. This is a common story – in one study of 400 police spouses, it was found that there is significant "spill-over" of stress from police onto their families (Alexander & Walker, 1996). The most stressful factors of police work that impacted spouses were the long work hours, the shift nature of the work, and the fact that leave time could be canceled at any moment for a police emergency. This stress proved to be too much for Bill's wife, and she left. What this means for his current state is that he is more socially isolated and less socially integrated than he would have been if he remained married. This in turn has significantly increased his risk of depression and suicidality (Motillon-Toudic et al., 2022; Van As et al., 2022).

In summary, both the conditions of his working life and the conditions of his retired life has set the scene for Bill's original presenting problem – depression and suicidality. Fortunately for Bill, as soon as he got some purpose back, along with some social connections, those issues resolved themselves. So what's next for Bill Hodges?

Move Over Depression – Here Comes Heart Disease

We can see a significant improvement in Bill's depressive symptoms and suicidality once he becomes fully enmeshed in his search for the Mr. Mercedes killer. Despite improvements to his mental well-being, his physical health remains problematic.

This is clearly demonstrated when Bill takes Jerome and Odell (Jerome's sweet Irish Setter) for an ice cream after Jerome has stopped by to look at Bill's computer. Bill is getting out of the house – he is walking, he is enjoying the company of others, he is sating his want of a strawberry ice cream. These are all things that would have been unfathomable in his earlier depressive state. It is what we would call behavioral activation – he is participating in acts that allow him to engage with others and participate in activities that he finds full of enjoyment and meaning (Kanter et al., 2010).

Clear improvement over Bill sitting among chip crumbs in his lounger, watching *Judge Judy*, and contemplating uses for his firearm. Yet he is not in the clear – as during the walk home from ice cream and Sherlocking, Bill struggles. He is losing his breath, and he can feel the extra pounds he has put on since retirement. What does this mean for a hard-boiled detective? Let's find out.

The Heart of Bill Hodges

Before we get into how Bill Hodges' 40 years as a cop, his retirement, his personality traits, and his exposure to stress impacted his cardiovascular health, let's just review what the heart and cardiovascular system are and do. The cardiovascular system, of course, includes your heart, but it also encompasses the blood and the blood vessels that transport that blood throughout the body. However, we could say that within this system, the most important part is the heart – as it is responsible for pumping blood to the lungs so that it can get oxygenated and then pump that oxygenated blood to the rest of the body (including the brain) and then bringing it back again.

Let's get more specific – have a look at Figure 5.1 – it shows exactly how the heart does this. When blood has just been through the body, providing oxygen-rich nutrients throughout, it returns to the heart via veins and the superior (from the upper body) and inferior (from the lower body) vena cava.[3] It enters the right atrium and flows into the right ventricle – which then pumps it through the pulmonary artery to the lungs. It is then reoxygenated and sent back to the heart via the pulmonary veins (to confuse you a bit, the pulmonary veins are the only veins that do have oxygenated blood). That blood then enters back into the heart via the left atrium into the left ventricle, then gets pumped out of the left ventricle into the aorta, and out to the rest of the body, starting the cycle all over again.

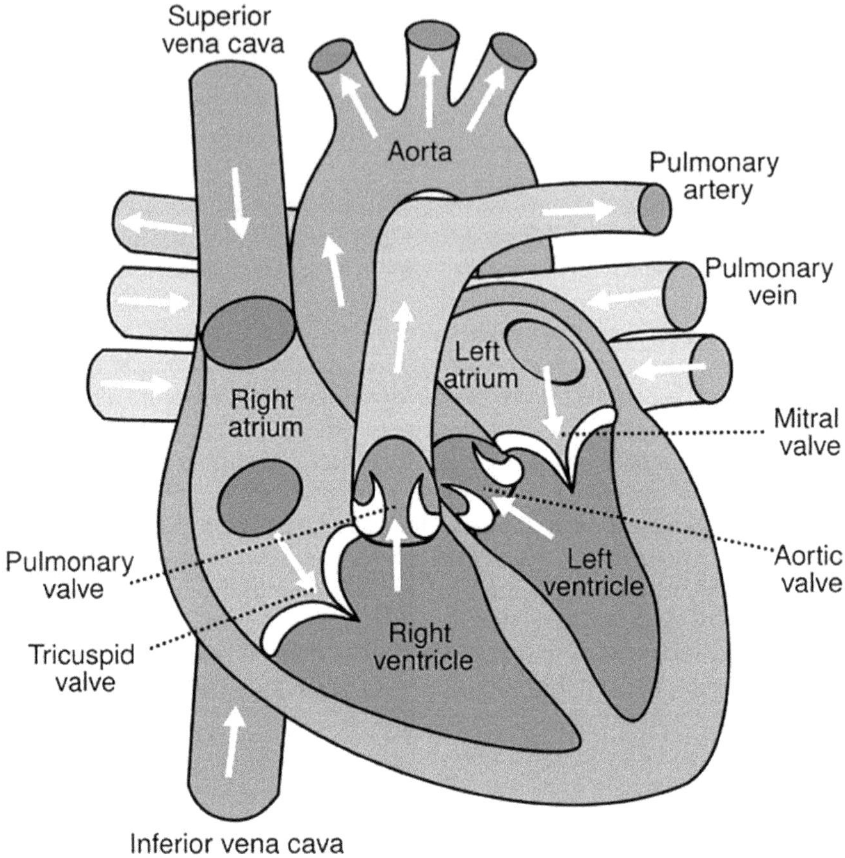

Figure 5.1 The Human Heart.

A few other things to know about the heart – we have a series of valves (tricuspid, pulmonary, mitral, and aortic), which prevents blood from flowing backward in the wrong direction. The important action within the heart that keeps this cycle going is the pumping I described occurring in the ventricles. This is what our blood pressure readings are measuring. The top number of our blood pressure reading refers to the systolic pressure – that is, how much pressure is being exerted by those ventricles when they are pushing the blood onto the atria through the ventricles. Diastolic pressure, or the bottom number, is the pressure when the heart is not pumping, but the ventricle is filling up with blood from the atria prior to being pumped out. That is why the bottom number is always lower than the top number – the top number is the action state, the bottom number is the resting state. A normal blood pressure would be around 120/80 mmHg.[4]

Hypertension occurs when you start seeing consistently high blood pressure readings.[5] Essential hypertension – where there is no single cause – was listed as one of Franz Alexander's Holy Seven of Psychosomatic Medicine that we discussed in Chapter 2. But in general, hypertension is caused by a variety of factors, including your genetics, your age, your diet and weight, physical activity, and so forth. This is why hypertension and the diseases that result from it are considered lifestyle diseases – those non-communicable diseases that were part of the epidemiological shift that occurred in the last century.

This brings us to cardiovascular disease (CVD). CVD is actually a blanket term for any of the diseases that impact the cardiovascular system – from strokes that impact the blood vessels and blood flow to the brain, to coronary heart disease (CHD) which impacts the arteries that provide blood to the heart itself. Let us think about CHD for a second, as this one may be important to Bill Hodge's diagnosis and prognosis.

Think back to the fact that a pumping action needs to occur in order for the blood to get through the heart to the lungs and then back out to the body. This pumping is done mostly by those thick muscles around the ventricles in Figure 5.1. Thus, those muscles are extremely important, and the arteries that supply blood to them in order for them to function are extremely important too. Those arteries that supply blood to the heart muscles are called coronary arteries – and when those become blocked or damaged – that is when big trouble ensues.

Big Trouble for Bill ⚠ [Spoiler Alert]

That big trouble is what happens to Bill, when *Mr. Mercedes* reaches its climax – when Bill, Holly, and Jerome race to thwart the bombing at the Mingo auditorium. Let's go through that day and see how CVD manifests itself for Bill – resulting in his (thankfully) non-fatal heart attack.

Deep into the pursuit, Bill starts to feel like he has pulled a muscle in his shoulder, though he actually has a sneaking suspicion it may be something a lot worse. What Bill is experiencing here is referred pain (Foreman et al., 2015). The pain in his shoulder is typical of how men experience cardiac pain – the pain from the heart is often "referred" out to other parts of the body due to complex interactions within the central and peripheral nervous system.

Next, after breaking into Brady's house and finding command central in his basement, he becomes "winded." He needs to take long breaths to try to regain his breathing. Multiple things are probably happening at this point – because his heart is not functioning properly, it is not pumping oxygenated blood to where it needs to go – including his lungs. If his lungs cannot function correctly, not only will he not be able to breathe in enough oxygen and breathe out enough carbon dioxide, he may also be experiencing pulmonary edema – where the lungs fill up with fluid because of decreased functioning.

Bill flat-out calls it while he is at the Mingo: "I'm having a heart attack." What he is referring to is a myocardial infarction (MI). "Myo" here refers to muscle, and "cardia" refers to the heart. The infarction refers to the death of tissue in the heart muscle. How did this occur? Remember when we discussed the importance of those coronary arteries that provide blood to the thick pumping muscles around the ventricles? When those become blocked, they can no longer provide oxygen to those muscles, and those muscles die. When those muscles die, they can no longer pump the blood to get oxygenated or to the rest of the body. Hence, the heart stops being able to do the life-sustaining activity it is meant to do.

What exactly happened? How did Bill's coronary arteries get to this point, where they could no longer provide oxygen-rich blood for his heart muscles? The main mechanism that leads to MI is atherosclerosis, which is when a bunch of substances build up in your coronary arteries, making them much narrower, and making it much more difficult for the blood to get through them to the heart muscle. From what we have read regarding Bill, I propose that there are four main biopsychosocial mechanisms that lead to his CVD (atherosclerosis) and ultimately his heart attack at the Mingo.

A Career of Vigilance

As mentioned in our discussion of depression and suicidality, the law enforcement profession comes with a lot of risks. One is that LEOs have higher CVD risk factors. Following LEOs and non-LEOs over a span of approximated seven years, Wright and colleagues (2011) found that LEOs had significantly higher systolic blood pressure, body mass index, waist circumference, and C-reactive protein – a marker of inflammation. These findings were repeated more recently by White et al. (2024), who found that LEOs had a higher mean body mass index compared to civilians, and they also had higher levels of IL-6, another inflammatory marker. This study went a step further and looked at levels of social vigilance among the two groups. LEOs had significantly higher total levels of social vigilance, which could be a potential link between law enforcement and CVD.

In another study that looked at over 100,000 police officers in Korea, researchers found that police officers had a significant increase in both developing CVD and in having acute MIs (Ki et al., 2024).

Is Bill Hodges Type A?

Of course, the nature of his work for 40 years has played a role in his physical health – but what about his personality? There is no doubt that Bill has severe CVD. For many decades, research focused on what types of personality could make a person more susceptible to CVD. The 1970s and 1980s saw a big focus on Type A personality as a potential driver of cardiovascular outcomes. Type A personality was first described by the cardiologists Rosenman and Friedman in the 1950s. A Type A person was someone who was quick to anger, who was extremely ambitious and competitive and who experienced constant time urgency. In both men and women, they found that those with more Type A characteristics had higher cholesterol, higher blood pressure, and a higher incidence of heart disease (Rosenman & Friedman, 1961).

Despite the dearth of research on Type A and heart disease that followed, two things began to happen – personality theorists started to believe that the Personality Type A vs Type B (the opposite of Type A) was too simplistic, and it started to emerge that only one aspect of Type A was truly predictive of cardiovascular outcomes – that is, hostility/anger. Many subsequent reviews and meta-analyses have shown a strong link between hostility and anger and a host of cardiovascular outcomes (Busch et al., 2017; Chida & Steptoe, 2009; Smith et al., 2004).

What about Bill Hodges? Would we consider him hostile? Prone to anger? Could this be a contributing factor, along with the nature of his job, and the stressful situations that he puts himself into? Let us look at one of the standard ways health psychologists measure hostility – the Cook–Medley Hostility Scale. The Cook–Medley started out as part of the Minnesota Multiphasic Personality Inventory and includes 50 true-false questions. Looking it over, there are a few questions that I know Bill Hodges would endorse, increasing his hostility score:

1 *I have often had to take orders from someone who did not know as much as I did.*
   It is his strong endorsement of this statement that causes Bill to go rogue in the first place, handling the Mr. Mercedes case himself after retiring from the police. He does not trust that the people who are now in charge of the case will do what needs to be done to get it solved, and so he bypasses the bureaucracy to get it done right.
2 *I think a great many people exaggerate their misfortunes in order to gain sympathy and the help of others.*
   I think this is demonstrated by Bill and Pete's early interactions with Olivia Trelawny, the owner of the hijacked Mercedes. During their first interrogation of Mrs. Trelawny, Bill notes with aggravation her focus on her own emotional turmoil – the fact that she will have to sell her beloved Mercedes, that she is tired, that she is the victim. He imagines himself slapping her across the face. As Bill states, "to… him – Mrs. T had just been a self-pitying rich lady who refused to accept her part in what happened." (King, 2014, p.71).
   Bill's immediate reaction toward Mrs. Trelawney is a good indication that his underlying, automatic thought process does lean toward hostility. Of course, later, after finding out more details about Olivia Trelawney from her sister, he rethinks this idea of her, but this logical overwriting of his original hostile interpretation of her is the exception that proves the rule.
3 *I would certainly enjoy beating a crook at his own game.*
   While Bill acknowledges the horror of the City Centre Massacre, he also thoroughly enjoys the idea of the chase. His mood immediately perks up when he receives the initial letter from Brady, not just because it gives him a newfound purpose, but because he gets back into a cat-and-mouse dynamic with a wily criminal. He is thrilled at sitting down with the letter – dissecting it for tells that he knows Brady thinks are "tricking" him. Bill picks up on the fact that Brady is using multiple red herrings to hide his writing style, and yet the incorporation of "perk" instead of "perp" is a spot he knows he can get him at. He even does this at the expense of the case, his own well-being, and legality.
4 *I have at times had to be rough with people who are rude or annoying.*
   There are many times that Bill Hodges is a little bit rougher than he has to be. Bill has a propensity to use more force than is probably warranted in certain situations. For example, after he has lunch with Pete in Lowtown, Bill notices

some bigger kids harassing a small kid. In a methodically slow saunter, he heads toward the melee. During the walk, he checks to make sure he has his "Happy Slapper" in his pocket – a sock filled with ball-bearings. He gives the big kids one chance to leave without incident, but they don't get the message. Bill proceeds to pummel one big kid in the neck with the sock (being sure to avoid the fatal area around the Adam's apple). Another big kid receives a powerful kick to the groin. As the two fall over in pain, the third one wisely makes his exit. It never crosses his mind NOT to be this rough in this situation, which is why I think this item from the Cook–Medley scale gets a "yes" for Bill.

A Lonely Life and Retirement

Bill's job, along with his hostility, probably had a significant impact on his social connections. While we briefly talked about his loneliness in retirement, and how that probably was a contributing factor to his depression and suicidality, we should also talk about it in terms of his general health. In particular, we should talk about his social integration (SI). I admit I am a bit biased when it comes to SI, as the majority of my PhD training was focused on how SI impacts health. SI refers to how many social roles and relationships one actively participates in (Crittenden & Cohen, 2024).

As is most pertinent to Bill Hodges, SI was first proposed as a concept by the French sociologist Emile Durkheim in the late 1800s. Durkheim was interested in factors associated with suicide. What he found were higher rates of suicide among the unmarried, as well as those with no children. When it came to suicide prevention, he considered roles such as being an employee, having a family, and being a part of a church, to be the most protective.

Even just looking at the work of a French sociologist from over a century ago, we can start to see where Bill is running into problems. In my investigations of SI and health (Crittenden et al., 2014, 2018), I generally look at the following social roles:

- Spouse (currently married)
- Parent (sees their child at least once a month)
- Other relative (sees their relative at least once a month)
- Friend (sees a friend at least once a month)
- Church member (attends religious service at least once a month)
- Club member (attends club at least once a month)
- Volunteer (volunteered for an organization over the past year)
- Employee (currently employed)

Thus, when you score someone on how socially integrated they are using this role-based measure, they receive a score between 0 and 8. Note that even if you have multiple friends or volunteer for multiple organizations – it still counts as only one role – you have the role of a friend or the role of a volunteer no matter how "much" of each you have. Figure 5.2 provides a graph of how researchers look at SI

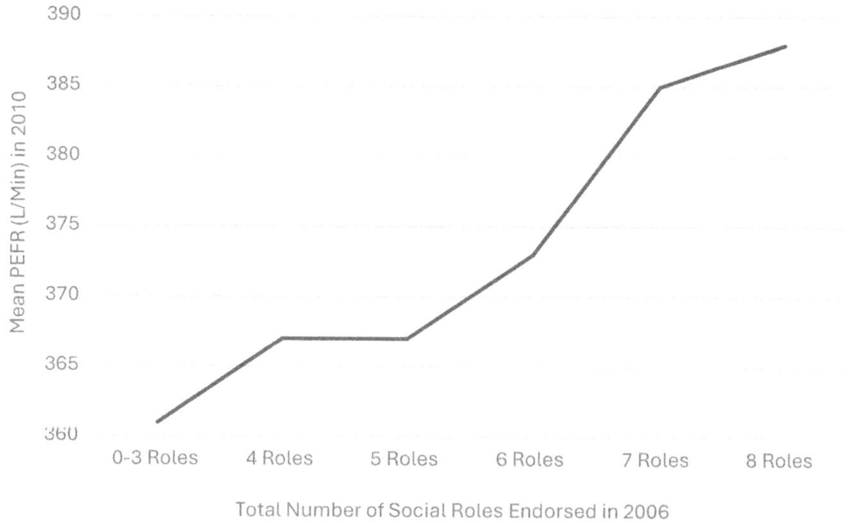

Figure 5.2 Association between Total Number of Social Roles and Average Peak Expiratory Flow Rate (PEFR).

in terms of health outcomes. On the bottom line (what we call the x-axis), you have the number of social roles someone said they participated in based on the above criteria, and then on the y-axis, you have their peak expiratory flow rate (PEFR). PEFR is a marker of how well their lungs are functioning. Higher PEFR means that you are able to get more air in and out of your lungs, which is always a good thing, especially for your heart.

Now, let's get back to Bill. We need to figure out his SI score when we first meet him. He is divorced, so he receives a 0 for having the marriage role. Bill does have an adult daughter named Allie who lives in San Francisco. While he hasn't seen her in person for many years, he mentions they do have "duty-calls" on Saturdays, so he would get a point here. Good news in the friend department too. Bill has spoken to Jerome at least in the last month about mowing the lawn, and he does consider him a friend, so he gets a point there. He does not discuss other relatives, any clubs, any volunteering, and he is definitely not a religious man – so zeros across the board here. Finally, his biggest trouble, retirement, means he is not currently employed, so another zero. This leaves Bill with a grand total SI score of two.

This opens Bill up to a whole host of problems, and as demonstrated by his trouble breathing while walking to get an ice cream with Jerome, his lung functioning is probably not the best. While we know we need the lungs to get oxygen to the heart and heart muscles – is there a connection between SI and CVD? In a recent systematic review by Chin and Cohen (2020), number of social roles were linked to multiple cardiovascular outcomes in numerous studies. For example, multiple studies among men found that the fewer social roles you had, the more likely you were to die from CVD. It was also found that fewer social roles were associated with poorer overall progression outcomes among those with CVD.

It looks like Bill's low SI number has put him at risk for CVD, and for that CVD to be fatal. But have no fear! As I will discuss later in this chapter, not only did Brady Hartsfield and his taunting letter give Bill purpose in life, but it upped his SI numbers – and thus may have prevented his heart attack from being fatal.

The Mingo Is the Last Straw – For Bill's Heart ⚠ [Spoiler Alert]

We have now considered the many preclinical risk factors that have been at play on Bill Hodges' heart. We will now take a quick look at what put that heart over the edge – the acute stressors of Brady's attempted attack on the Mingo auditorium.

Yes, long-term exposure to vigilance, hostility, and loneliness made Bill's heart weak. The continued high blood pressure caused Bill's heart to work harder, as well as his arteries. The constant pressure going through the arteries weakened them, and also probably caused a build-up of plague and other detritus that significantly narrowed the passages. Thus, blood flow was being restricted, and blood was not getting to places it needed to go. Importantly, if this narrowing of the arteries occurred in the coronary arteries, the blood wouldn't get to the heart muscles. Everything was set up and ready to go off at a moment's provocation.

That provocation was the fact that Brady Hartsfield was strapped with a wheelchair full of explosives and shrapnel, and was currently in the Mingo auditorium, enjoying a boy band, and getting ready to blow himself up. Knowing this and having a short amount of time to try and stop the death and dismemberment of hundreds of preteen girls is what I would call a significant acute stressor. And this acute stressor is the spark that lights the kindling of all of Bill's pre-existing conditions.

Multiple things could have happened at this point of high threat for Bill. First, we know for sure that he probably had a significant "fight or flight" response, and this in turn caused his sympathetic–adreno-medullary axis to release a whole lot of epinephrine (adrenaline) and norepinephrine. The result – Bill's heart rate and blood pressure shot up rapidly, putting an additional strain on an already weak heart. This fight of flight reaction can also significantly increase inflammatory reactions throughout the body, which would further narrow his coronary arteries. If there was a build-up of plague in those arteries, this increased pressure and inflammation could cause the plague to break apart and clog the arteries – preventing blood flow altogether.

All of this could lead to a reduction or stoppage of blood to the heart, leading the heart muscle to die – the infarct. For Bill, this all happened over several hours – things probably became progressively worse as his heart was less and less able to do what it needed to do as muscle tissue died. But it took that initial extreme fight or flight response to get the process rolling. Since the threat did not resolve itself right away, Bill was just repeatedly awash in the adrenaline and noradrenaline that eventually exhausted his system. The only way for him to survive at that point was to get medical assistance. Luckily, he gets to the hospital and the condition is treated before further damage can be done. The damage is significant though – Bill will need a pacemaker[6] for the rest of his life to help assist his significantly weakened heart.

Bill Dodges Bullet – This Time

Thankfully for us Bill Hodges fans out there, Bill survived his heart attack and even used it as a cue to action to get healthier. One of the things that probably helped him do this was the increase in social connections that resulted from his off-the-books investigation of the Mercedes killer. If you remember, during his initial six months of retirement, Bill had scored a two on the SI scale. At the end of *Mr. Mercedes*, and the beginning of *Finders Keepers*, we can probably bump that up a few points. His detective work has become official, so he gets a point for employee. While this may not be official, I do believe that Bill sees Holly, Janey's cousin, as his relative through her, so I'm going to give him a point for "other relative." I'm also going to give him a point for volunteering, since I think he would consider going to visit a comatose Brady in the hospital as a generous donation of his time.

Not only has Bill upped his SI score, but I think the number of people in each role category has increased significantly, increasing his overall level of social connections. This is extremely good for Bill as it has been found that the more social connections, and thus social support, one has, the more likely one is to remain alive six months after MI (Mookadam & Arthur, 2004). Bill is able, with the help of those around him, to go on a strict diet – no junk food, mostly salad and water. Holly is the one who keeps him in check and is a great example why social support is so important.

⚠ **[Spoiler Alert]**

End of Watch – *Cancer*

Bill is feeling great – until he isn't. In the last book, *End of Watch*, Bill has become a bit more lax in making sure he goes to all his health checkups. One of the reasons for this is that while his heart is good, he is starting to experience pain in other areas of his body. He is experiencing some pretty consistent stomach pain, and this is causing him some health care hesitancy:

> Like most elderly guys he knows, he doesn't like doctors' offices. He is always afraid they're going to find not just something wrong but something *really* wrong.
>
> (King, 2016, p.16)

This is called delay behavior. In this case, it sounds like Bill my be avoiding what he feels is inevitable – and the longer he delays, the more time he has before his life is taken over by another medical crisis. Eventually, the nagging pain and the nagging Holly get him to go see a doctor. Finally, he gets the results he was dreading – he has pancreatic cancer, and it is rather far into its progression. It has spread to his liver, and he has about a year to live – maybe two. But we won't fault Bill for the fact that they caught it so late – pancreatic cancer is one of those cancers that is very hard to detect early, which is why it is so deadly (Halbrook et al., 2023).

Bill being Bill, he downplays his diagnosis (it's just an ulcer) to everyone and is not sure if he would like to undergo the treatment. There are many reasons why he may not want treatment – he worries that the treatment will be worse than the disease itself, and this plays into worry about how his quality of life will be impacted. He may also just feel that with such a progressive and deadly form of cancer, there isn't much hope to be placed in treatment.

How did Bill get to this point? It is interesting to note that many of the same factors that put him at risk for CVD also put him at risk for cancer. Multiple studies have found that being in law enforcement leads to higher rates of cancer morbidity and mortality (Heikkinen et al., 2023; Violanti et al., 2021). The same association is found for social isolation and loneliness (Wang et al., 2023).

I will not say too much about what happens next. Just know that while the struggles that Bill was tortured with in the beginning of the series were replaced by CVD and cancer, they were also replaced with love, friendship, and a sense of purpose that solved many a mystery, as well as saved many a life.

The Bill Hodges Trilogy

Mr. Mercedes

Novel: King, S. (2014). *Mr. Mercedes: A Novel*. Scribner.
Audiobook: King, S. (2014). *Mr. Mercedes* (W. Patton, Narr.) [Audiobook]. Simon & Schuster Audio.
TV Series: Kelley, D. E. (Executive Producer). (2017–2019). *Mr. Mercedes* [TV series]. Audience Network; Sonar Entertainment.

Finders Keepers

Novel: King, S. (2015). *Finders Keepers*. Scribner.
Audiobook: King, S. (2015). *Finders Keepers* (W. Patton, Narr.) [Audiobook]. Simon & Schuster Audio.

End of Watch

Novel: King, S. (2016). *End of Watch*. Scribner.
Audiobook: King, S. (2016). *End of Watch* (W. Patton, Narr.) [Audiobook]. Simon & Schuster Audio.

Further Explorations

1 There are several self-report measurements for "Purpose in Life." The most frequently used is the Purpose in Life Scale (PIL; Crumbaugh & Maholick, 1964). In addition, there is the Life Engagement Test (LET; Scheier et al., 2006),[7] and

the Meaning in Life Questionnaire (MLQ; Steger et al., 2006). If you do a quick search on the internet, you should be able to find the measurements. Fill out the questionnaires as if you were Bill Hodges at the beginning of *Mr. Mercedes*, and at the end (or at the beginning of *Finders Keepers*). How did you score? What significant changes did you see? What could account for those changes?

2 Take a look at the full Cook–Medley scale – you can easily search for it. What other items do you think Bill Hodges would endorse? Provide an example or examples that make you think he would answer in that way. Does this make him more or less susceptible to poor cardiovascular outcomes?

Notes

1 We discuss the DSM-5 in more detail in Chapter 9, where we discuss sleep and insomnia.

2 A "beat cop" is a police officer who patrols – they are the frontline, patrolling areas, responding to emergencies, and making their presence known among the community – in order to prevent criminal activity and create a sense of safety. We can assume that this is where Bill started his law enforcement career, eventually moving into the behind-the-scenes role as a detective.

3 It is important to note that anatomy and physiology textbooks usually always show our veins and the vena cava as blue, in order to indicate that this is the return pathway of de-oxygenated blood. The blood itself is not blue – blood is always red in color.

4 mmHg stands for millimeters of mercury. This is because in the early days, blood pressure was measured by how high the pressure of your blood could shoot some mercury up a tube. Of course, we don't use that measurement method anymore, but we still use the terminology.

5 There is also a condition known as White Coat Hypertension, which does not occur consistently, but only when someone is in a health care setting. This is discussed more in Chapter 8, as it relates to Stu Redman in *The Stand.*

6 The pacemaker will provide electrical signals to make sure the heart beats at a steady pace.

7 The Life Engagement Test, or LET, was made possible by the Pittsburgh Mind-Body Center (PMBC) that we discussed in Chapter 2.

Bibliography

Alexander, D. A., & Walker, L. G. (1996). The perceived impact of police work on police officer's spouses and families. *Stress Medicine*, *12*(4), 239–246. https://doi.org/10.1002/(SICI)1099-1700(199610)12:4<239::AID-SMI707>3.0.CO;2-3

American Psychiatric Association. (2013). *Diagnostic and statistical manual of mental disorders* (5th ed.). https://doi.org/10.1176/appi.books.9780890425596

Bonnewyn, A., Shah, A., Bruffaerts, R., & Demyttenaere, K. (2014). Are gender and life attitudes associated with the wish to die in older psychiatric and somatic inpatients? An explorative study. *International Psychogeriatrics*, *26*(10), 1693–1702. https://doi.org/10.1017/S1041610214000957

Bureau of Labor Statistics, U.S. Department of Labor. *Occupational outlook handbook, police and detectives*, from https://www.bls.gov/ooh/protective-service/police-and-detectives.htm (visited August 28, 2025).

Busch, L. Y., Pössel, P., & Valentine, J. C. (2017). Meta-analyses of cardiovascular reactivity to rumination: A possible mechanism linking depression and hostility to cardiovascular disease. *Psychological Bulletin*, *143*(12), 1378. https://doi.org/10.1037/bul0000119

Chida, Y., & Steptoe, A. (2009). The association of anger and hostility with future coronary heart disease: A meta-analytic review of prospective evidence. *Journal of the American College of Cardiology*, *53*(11), 936–946. https://doi.org/10.1016/j.jacc.2008.11.044

Chin, B., & Cohen, S. (2020). Review of the association between number of social roles and cardiovascular disease: Graded or threshold effect? *Psychosomatic Medicine*, *82*(5), 471–486. https://doi.org/10.1097/PSY.0000000000000809

Chopko, B. A., Palmieri, P. A., & Adams, R. E. (2013). Associations between police stress and alcohol use: Implications for practice. *Journal of Loss and Trauma*, *18*(5), 482–497. https://doi.org/10.1080/15325024.2012.719340Crittenden, C. N., & Cohen, S. (2024). Social integration. In F. Maggino (Ed.), *Encyclopedia of quality of life and well-being research* (pp. 6601–6605). Springer International Publishing. https://doi.org/10.1007/s978-3-031-17299-1_2769

Crittenden, C. N., Murphy, M. L., & Cohen, S. (2018). Social integration and age-related decline in lung function. *Health Psychology*, *37*(5), 472–480. https://doi.org/10.1037/hea0000592

Crittenden, C. N., Pressman, S. D., Cohen, S., Janicki-Deverts, D., Smith, B. W., & Seeman, T. E. (2014). Social integration and pulmonary function in the elderly. *Health Psychology*, *33*(6), 535–543. https://doi.org/10.1037/hea0000029

Crumbaugh, J. C., & Maholick, L. T. (1964). An experimental study in existentialism: The psychometric approach to Frankl's concept of noogenic neurosis. *Journal of Clinical Psychology*, *20*(2), 200–207.

Foreman, R. D., Garrett, K. M., & Blair, R. W. (2015). Mechanisms of cardiac pain. *Comprehensive Physiology*, *5*(2), 929–960. https://doi.org/10.1002/cphy.c140032

Halbrook, C. J., Lyssiotis, C. A., di Magliano, M. P., & Maitra, A. (2023). Pancreatic cancer: Advances and challenges. *Cell*, *186*(8), 1729–1754. https://doi.org/10.1016/j.cell.2023.02.014

Heikkinen, S., Demers, P. A., Hansen, J., Jakobsen, J., Kjaerheim, K., Lynge, E., … & Pukkala, E. (2023). Incidence of cancer among Nordic police officers. *International Journal of Cancer*, *152*(6), 1124–1136. https://doi.org/10.1002/ijc.34311

Kanter, J. W., Manos, R. C., Bowe, W. M., Baruch, D. E., Busch, A. M., & Rusch, L. C. (2010). What is behavioral activation? A review of the empirical literature. *Clinical Psychology Review*, *30*(6), 608–620. https://doi.org/10.1016/j.cpr.2010.04.001 [psycnet.apa.org]

Ki, M., Lapierre, S., Gim, B., Hwang, M., Kang, M., Dargis, L., … & Mishara, B. (2024). A systematic review of psychosocial protective factors against suicide and suicidality among older adults. *International Psychogeriatrics*, *36*(5), 346–370. https://doi.org/10.1017/S104161022300443X

Kim, E. S., Chen, Y., Nakamura, J. S., Ryff, C. D., & VanderWeele, T. J. (2022). Sense of purpose in life and subsequent physical, behavioral, and psychosocial health: An outcome-wide approach. *American Journal of Health Promotion*, *36*(1), 137–147. https://doi.org/10.1177/08901171211038545

Kim, E. S., Delaney, S. W., & Kubzansky, L. D. (2019). Sense of purpose in life and cardiovascular disease: Underlying mechanisms and future directions. *Current Cardiology Reports*, *21*(11), 135. https://doi.org/10.1007/s11886-019-1222-9King, S. (2014). *Mr. Mercedes*. Scribner. https://www.amazon.com/dp/B00GEEB0N6

King, S. (2015). *Finders Keepers*. Scribner. https://www.amazon.com/dp/B00P42WROG

King, S. (2016). *End of Watch*. Scribner. https://www.amazon.com/dp/B00P42WROG

Klösch, G., Zeitlhofer, J., & Ipsiroglu, O. (2022). Revisiting the concept of vigilance. *Frontiers in Psychiatry*, *13*, 874757. https://doi.org/10.3389/fpsyt.2022.874757

Li, W., Ye, X., Zhu, D., & He, P. (2021). The longitudinal association between retirement and depression: A systematic review and meta-analysis. *American Journal of Epidemiology, 190*(10), 2220–2230. https://doi.org/10.1093/aje/kwab125

Magnavita, N., Chirico, F., Garbarino, S., & Ciprani, F. (2024). Stress, sleep, and cardiovascular risk in police officers: A scoping review. *Journal of Health and Social Sciences, 9*(1), 9–23. https://doi.org/10.19204/2024/STRS1 [publires.unicatt.it]

Mehta, P. K., Sharma, A., Bremner, J. D., & Vaccarino, V. (2022). Mental stress-induced myocardial ischemia. *Current Cardiology Reports, 24*(12), 2109–2120. https://doi.org/10.1007/s11886-022-01821-2Mookadam, F., & Arthur, H. M. (2004). Social support and its relationship to morbidity and mortality after acute myocardial infarction: Systematic overview. *Archives of Internal Medicine, 164*(14), 1514–1518. https://doi.org/10.1001/archinte.164.14.1514

Motillon-Toudic, C., Walter, M., Séguin, M., Carrier, J. D., Berrouiguet, S., & Lemey, C. (2022). Social isolation and suicide risk: Literature review and perspectives. *European Psychiatry, 65*(1), e65. https://doi.org/10.1192/j.eurpsy.2022.2320

Odone, A., Gianfredi, V., Vigezzi, G. P., Amerio, A., Ardito, C., d'Errico, A., … & Costa, G. (2021). Does retirement trigger depressive symptoms? A systematic review and meta-analysis. *Epidemiology and Psychiatric Sciences, 30*, e77. https://doi.org/10.1017/S2045796021000627

Reker, G. T. (1992). *Manual of the Life Attitude Profile–Revised.* Student Psychologists Press.

Rosenman, R. H., & Friedman, M. (1961). Association of specific behavior pattern in women with blood and cardiovascular findings. *Circulation, 24*(5), 1173–1184. https://doi.org/10.1161/01.CIR.24.5.1173

Scheier, M. F., Wrosch, C., Baum, A., Cohen, S., Martire, L. M., Matthews, K. A., … & Zdaniuk, B. (2006). The life engagement test: Assessing purpose in life. *Journal of Behavioral Medicine, 29*(3), 291–298. https://doi.org/10.1007/s10865-005-9044-1

Smith, T. W., Glazer, K., Ruiz, J. M., & Gallo, L. C. (2004). Hostility, anger, aggressiveness, and coronary heart disease: An interpersonal perspective on personality, emotion, and health. *Journal of Personality, 72*(6), 1217–1270. https://doi.org/10.1111/j.1467-6494.2004.00296.x

Steger, M. F., Frazier, P., Oishi, S., & Kaler, M. (2006). The meaning in life questionnaire: Assessing the presence of and search for meaning in life. *Journal of Counseling Psychology, 53*(1), 80. https://doi.org/10.1037/0022-0167.53.1.80

Van As, B. A. L., Imbimbo, E., Franceschi, A., Menesini, E., & Nocentini, A. (2022). The longitudinal association between loneliness and depressive symptoms in the elderly: A systematic review. *International Psychogeriatrics, 34*(7), 657–669. https://doi.org/10.1017/S1041610221000399

Violanti, J. M., Gu, J. K., Charles, L. E., Fekedulegn, D., & Andrew, M. E. (2021). Dying for the job: Police mortality, 1950–2018. *Policing: An International Journal, 44*(6), 1168–1187. https://doi.org/10.1108/PIJPSM-06-2021-0087

Wang, F., Gao, Y., Han, Z., Yu, Y., Long, Z., Jiang, X., … & Zhao, Y. (2023). A systematic review and meta-analysis of 90 cohort studies of social isolation, loneliness and mortality. *Nature Human Behaviour, 7*(8), 1307–1319. https://doi.org/10.1038/s41562-023-01617-6

White, S. C., Ruiz, J. M., Allison, M., Uchino, B. N., Smith, T. W., Taylor, D. J., ... & Smyth, J. M. (2024). Cardiovascular risk, social vigilance, and stress profiles of male law enforcement officers versus civilians. *Health Psychology Open, 11*, 1–10. https://doi.org/https://doi.org/10.1177/20551029241244723

Wirth, M., Vena, J. E., Smith, E. K., Bauer, S. E., Violanti, J., & Burch, J. (2013). The epidemiology of cancer among police officers. *American Journal of Industrial Medicine*, *56*(4), 439–453. https://doi.org/10.1002/ajim.22145

Wright, B. R., Barbosa-Leiker, C., & Hoekstra, T. (2011). Law enforcement officer versus non–law enforcement officer status as a longitudinal predictor of traditional and emerging cardiovascular risk factors. *Journal of Occupational and Environmental Medicine*, *53*(7), 730–734. https://doi.org/10.1097/JOM.0b013e318220c2da

6 Plot Development

The Bigger Picture of Health Influence

The Horror of Society

The Running Man[1] was published by Stephen King in 1982 under the pseudonym Richard Bachman. Other books by Bachman include *Thinner*, which we discussed in Chapter 4, *The Long Walk*, and the now out-of-print *Rage*,[2] *Roadwork*, *The Regulators*, and *Blaze*. When comparing Bachman novels to King novels, I feel that King finds the horrors in the supernatural, which can be defeated, whereas Bachman finds them in society, which can be a much harder foe to defeat. Bachman shows us how real-world horrors, which stem from individuals and the higher order structures in which they live, come to be.

Enter *The Running Man* (see Box 6.1), a story about a dystopian world in which an authoritarian government controls everything – from the distribution of "new money" to the types of marriages you can have, to selective healthcare accessibility. The government, aka The Network, also controls the flow of information through the Free-Vees, government-controlled televisions that everyone is required to have.

Box 6.1 *The Running Man*

Like *Thinner*, *The Running Man* was published under Stephen King's pseudonym, Richard Bachman, in 1982.

The book actually takes place in the same year that I am writing this book, 2025. Things in America are going even worse in this dystopian 2025 than they are going now. The story follows Ben Richards – a desperate man in desperate times. The desperate times refer to the fact that the United States has seen its economy tank, the climate is in ruins, and a totalitarian regime has taken control. The desperate man refers to the fact that Ben Richards and his wife Sheila have a 16-month-old daughter, Cathy, who is extremely sick. They cannot afford the life-saving medication Cathy needs, and Sheila has resorted to prostitution to get what money she can.

Ben himself is a bit of a hot-head, anti-establishment type, and has been out of work for some time. Wanting to right this wrong, and return to supporting

DOI: 10.4324/9781003495994-6

his family, he opts to volunteer for the Games Network. The Games Network is a television station, run by the government, that airs on government-provided televisions called Free-Vees. These are propaganda tools, and an important part of the propaganda is the airing of violent game shows. Here, people desperate for money voluntarily participate in games like "Treadmill to Bucks" – where people with heart conditions can earn money by staying on a treadmill as long as possible – before they collapse or die.

⚠ **[Spoiler Alert]** Despite Sheila's misgivings, Ben undergoes the intense screening process at the Games Network headquarters, and is chosen for the most popular game – "The Running Man". After being declared public enemy number one in front of the entire Free Vee viewing audience, he is given a 12-hour head start before he is tracked down by trained "Hunters." For every hour that he evades capture, he wins $100 for himself and his family. He also receives $100 for any law enforcement officer or Hunter he kills. If he can make it 30 days without being caught, he will win $1 billion.

On the flip side, the public is offered incentives – cash payments – for verified sighting of Ben Richards. They are also provided with a false narrative on who Ben Richards is, and how his capture is a patriotic imperative. This makes it very hard for Ben to trust anyone he may come in contact with on his "run" – but luckily, there are enough people out there disillusioned by the government and the current state of the world, that with their help, he becomes to longest-evading running man in the history of the game.

Through his flight from the hunters, Ben becomes even more enlightened on how the rest of the US is living, from the derelict conditions of the Boston YMCA to the polluted air, making those in certain poverty-stricken neighborhoods susceptible to lung cancer, even at the young age of five. He also sees how much the Free Vee, and the constant feed of propaganda, has distracted most of the country from seeing what a truly totalitarian state it has become. Yet Ben Richards does not seem to be falling quietly into their propaganda machine – with each evasion of "The Running Man" hunters, he seems to gather public support, with those of the lowest classes seeing his plight as a rallying cry.

In the end, through a series of desperate maneuvers, Ben manufactures an ending to "The Running Man" that no one saw coming. An end that is hopefully a new beginning for all the people that the Games Network, and the government, have so gleefully taken advantage of for years.

The Running Man's main plot stems from a health concern – the health of Ben Richard's daughter, Cathy, who has a severe case of pneumonia. Healthcare is not easily accessible to most people, especially those who don't make enough "new money" (old money is floating around but is mostly useless). Yet the availability of medicine and doctors is not the only thing that is impacting Cathy's health. We have the fact that her dad had to quit his job just to be able to have her, as the chemicals he was exposed to at work significantly impacted his fertility. Her family is also considered low socioeconomic status (SES), that is, they are of low income, low education, and low occupational status. They also live in a neighborhood overrun by violence, as well as rats (what we would call a vector of disease). The nutrition that they can afford is "greasy pizza wedges and government pill-commodities" (King, 2012, p.32). This is a multi-pronged attack on the health and wellbeing of the Richards family, and it is a great illustration of a key theory in health psychology – the ecological model

Bronfenbrenner's Ecological Model

The ecological model was first proposed by the psychologist Urie Bronfenbrenner (1977) to describe the multiple systems and environments that a human is exposed to as it goes through key developmental stages. Bronfenbrenner really felt that looking at how children develop by seeing what happens in laboratory settings, under manufactured conditions, was highly limiting. If you wanted to really see

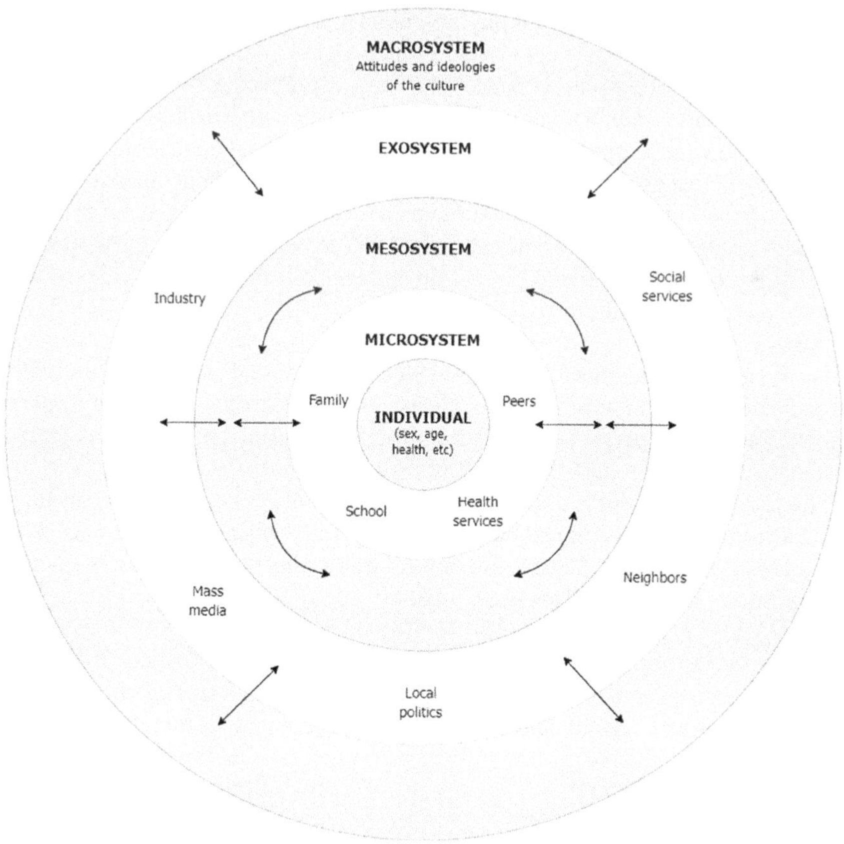

Figure 6.1 Bronfenbrenner's Ecological Model of Human Development.

how children develop, you needed to look at the entire world that surrounds them and impacts them on a regular basis.

Figure 6.1 provides a very simple sketch of what this would look like. In the middle, you have the child, or the individual. These are the things specific to the person that may be impacting their development, or as what we are concerned with – their health. This includes age at the time we are considering, sex/gender, underlying genetic makeup, including health markers such as current immune system functioning, etc.

Outside of this, you have the microsystem – the systems that are closest to you in both physical and emotional proximity. This includes your family, your friends, the school you attend, and the adults and peers you interact with there, the health services you (hopefully) have regular access to, and other close and frequently used social structures – like church.

Heading outward, you then have the mesosystem. According to Bronfenbrenner, the mesosystem is how those structures in your microsystem relate to each other – how parents participate in school, how schools may interrelate with health services, and how churches may impact families. In essence, these are the interactions between the components of the individual's microsystem.

Next, we have the exosystem, where other higher social structures start to be included in mesosystem interactions. What was important to Bronfenbrenner here was that these are systems that may not have direct contact with the individual at the center, but what happens within them has a direct impact on that individual. The intricacies of local government may never come into physical contact with the individual, and the individual may never have an awareness that they even exist – but the decisions they make have a direct impact on the individual. For example – does the local government decide to protect the green space near the individual's home so that a park can be built for the child to enjoy, or do they opt to sell it for industrial purposes?

Lastly, we have the macrosystem – which is the most distant to the individual, but may determine how the micro-, meso-, and exosystems are able to operate. Macrosystems incorporate important and all-encompassing cultural beliefs, including the ideologies that control society as a whole.

The ecological model is used to guide a plethora of research on how our micro- and macroenvironments impact our health, especially when it comes to health disparities (Reifsnider et al., 2005). When we speak of health disparities, we will use the definition put forth by Braveman in 2006:

> Health disparities/inequalities are potential avoidable differences in health (or in health risks that policy can influence) between groups of people who are more and less advantaged socially; these differences systematically place socially disadvantaged groups at further disadvantage on health.
>
> (Braveman, 2006, p.180)

We are going to stick with Bronfenbrenner here and look at the developmental health aspects of the ecological model on the two children we meet in *The Running Man* – Ben Richard's daughter, Cathy, and Cassie, the sister of Bradley

Throckmorton, who helps Ben escape Boston. Each girl is experiencing a health crisis, and each crisis can be tied to the ecological structure of the dystopian society in which they live.

The Individuals

First, let's take a look at each of these individuals who are suffering such significant impacts of the environment in which they live.

Catherine "Cathy" Sarah Richards

Cathy Richards is an 18-month-old White female. She is an only child, and lives with her parents in a small non-heated apartment in the impoverished Midwest neighborhood of Co-Op City. Co-Op City is overrun with garbage and rats. There is no visible police presence, and the city consists of mostly closed down shops and parking lots. The air in Co-Op City is "sulfurous and thick" (King, 2012, p.7) on more days than not. Her parents are uneducated and unemployed and receive minimal government benefits ($20 a week in old money, and government nutritional pills). To make up for their financial shortcomings, Cathy's mother Sheila will often fall back on prostitution to make ends meet.

Healthwise, Cathy has pneumonia. Chances are her diagnosis would be community-acquired pneumonia, which simply means she acquired it outside the hospital setting (Vaughn et al., 2024). Pneumonia is the infectious disease that kills the most people in the United States each year, and it affects the lower respiratory tract. Symptoms include difficulty breathing and cough, along with high fever – all of which Cathy is suffering from. Unfortunately, the only healthcare the Richardses have access to is a midwife practicing in unsanitary conditions, and any black market penicillin they can find.

Cassie Throckmorton

Cassie Throckmorton is a five-year-old Black female who lives in an impoverished neighborhood of Boston. It has many of the same characteristics of Co-Op City, including highly polluted air. She lives with her mother and two older brothers, one of which is involved in a street gang called "The Stabbers." Similar to the Richards, no one is able to work, and they resort to illegal activities to get the money to make ends meet.

Cassie has been diagnosed with lung cancer, which has spread to her throat and digestive system. Medication can only be purchased when the sporadic payments for various illegal activities come in. While lung cancer is the leading cause of cancer deaths around the world, it is usually a disease of older (65+ years old) males (CDC, 2025). Cassie's symptoms include chronic and debilitating pain in her chest and abdomen, extreme tiredness and body weakness, and constant coughing.

Both Cathy and Cassie are suffering from significant respiratory diseases, which indicate that the ecological factors around them impacting their health have to do

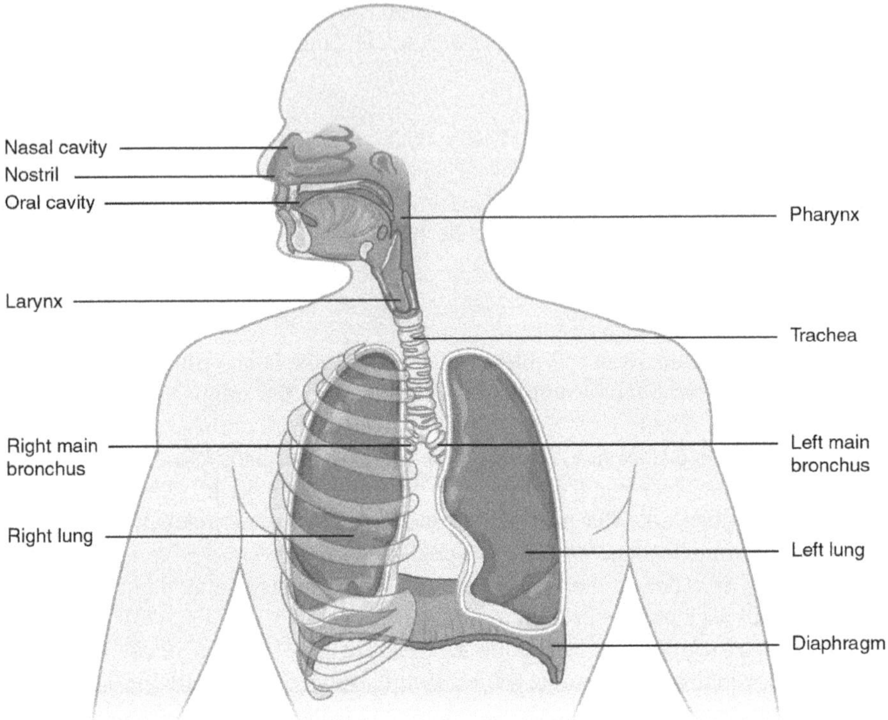

Figure 6.2 The Respiratory System.

with air and breathing. Before we go over the ecological factors by level, I think it is worth doing a quick overview of the respiratory system. In Chapter 5, when discussing Bill Hodges and the trouble with cardiovascular disease, I mentioned the importance of oxygen-rich blood getting to the body. How the heart is able to do this is via the lungs – the organs that are able to take oxygen and deliver it to the body via blood, and to remove the carbon dioxide byproduct. Let's talk about how this happens.

Take a look at Figure 6.2. You breath in, and in doing so, the air goes through your nose, mouth, or both. This is actually part of both the respiratory system and the immune system – for example, the hairs and mucus of the nose are going to act like a first line of defense filter – making sure no foreign matter gets in. The next stop is your throat, or pharynx, and then your voice box (larynx), and finally, the air enters your trachea, which is commonly referred to as your windpipe. At the bottom, the trachea creates a Y shape, splitting itself into a left bronchus for the left lung, and a right bronchus for the right lung.

Once the air gets into the lungs via the bronchi, it starts traveling down tubes that get progressively smaller, called bronchioles. Eventually, they end in the sac-like structures you see represented in Figure 6.3. These are the alveoli, and it is here where the oxygen – carbon dioxide transfer occurs. You can see that around

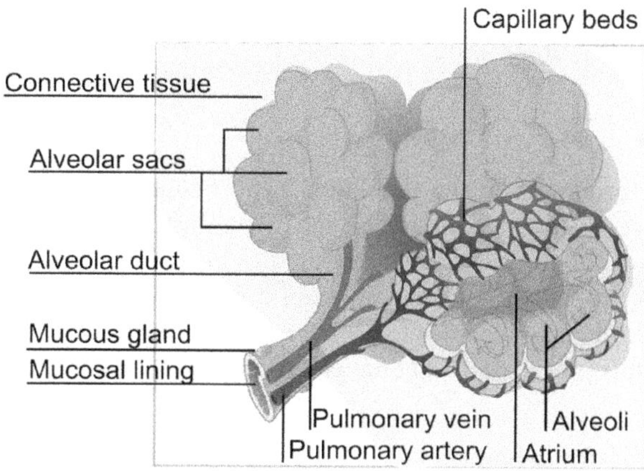

Figure 6.3 Alveolus of the Respiratory System.

the alveoli are blood vessels – here is where the oxygen goes through the wall of the sacs to enrich the blood (which will go back to the heart to be pumped to the rest of the body) and where the carbon dioxide waste-rich blood from the body passes on the carbon dioxide through the wall into the sacs so that it then can be expelled when we breathe out.

As you can guess, a lot depends on the airways remaining open and clean. How efficient our lungs are at getting oxygen to the rest of the body also depends on how much of the air we take in is actually oxygen. Think back to our discussion in Chapter 2 about miasma theory – the idea that the air we breathe in was filled with many other things besides oxygen – that made us sick with diseases like the plague. While the diseases that people attributed to miasma were found to be caused by other things (rodent vectors, contaminated drinking water) – the idea that the air which we breathe could have a huge impact on our health is very much an important health factor. And this is very evident throughout *The Running Man.*

It is clear throughout the book that the dystopian Co-Op City, as well as the Boston "ghettos," are overwhelmed by pollution. The air quality in these areas is so bad that the government has stopped publishing the air-pollution counts, in hopes that the people will just "forget." Of course, Bradley and his gang haven't forgotten, and they use their stolen library card (you can only get a library card if you have a guaranteed income of 5,000 new dollars a year) to get the info to build their own pollution counter.

The pollution stems mostly from industry, and at one point, especially when weather was apt to make pollution counts worse, industries had to shut down until the weather shifted. A revised congressional law, however, did away with those requirements, so that industrial pollution output is a 24/7 occurrence, especially in the poorer neighborhoods that are downstream. Of course, why are the poorer neighborhoods always downstream – because the people who can afford to move away do, and they use their money to make sure laws are passed to keep their new neighborhoods pollution-free. Who is left are the people who cannot afford to move away, or advocate for themselves on a government level. This is the lot of Ben, Bradley, Cathy, and Cassie.

Individual Level

We have described some of the individual factors that each of the girls possess. Both of them seem too young, and of the wrong sex, for the diseases they are battling. It seems the individual factors may not be as important here as the other levels. There is probably one exception, and that is the fact that Cassie is a racial minority. Since this is not a risk factor that each of them shares, I will discuss the particular risk this puts Cassie in at the end of this chapter.

Microsystem Level and Mesosystem

On the microsystem level, you have the family and the family environment as contributors to the individual's health and development. In one way, you could see how the family environment (interacting with exosystem level phenomena) impacts both Cathy's and Cassie's lungs – and that is through cigarette smoking.

Both Ben Richards and Bradley Throckmorton smoke – and they smoke indoors due to the dangers present in their impoverished and violent neighborhoods. This, of course, causes significant secondhand smoke dangers for those around them – especially the young children with developing lungs who are in their care. This leaves us with two questions – (1) Why are they smoking to begin with? (2) And what exact risk does it put Cathy and Cassie under?

Ben and Bradley would be considered low SES – as they occupy some of the lowest positions in this dystopian society – they do not have jobs, so they do not make money, and, in the case of Bradley, his race puts him in an even lowered position. Research suggests that smoking is more likely to become a habit when started in adolescence, and low SES adolescents are more often exposed to parents and peers who smoke, and are less able to ignore peer pressure (Hiscock et al., 2012) They also tend not to understand the dangers inherent in smoking, and they also have more cigarette availability in their low SES neighborhoods than what is available in high SES areas. Thus, SES is associated with higher rates of starting smoking. It is also associated with higher rates of relapse when one is trying to kick the habit. We know that lower SES is associated with higher exposures to stress, and an increased likelihood of being anxious or depressed, which in turn leads to more low SES individuals returning to smoking after they have tried to quit.

Lower SES is also associated with secondhand smoke exposure – or what we call environmental tobacco smoke (ETS). In one recent study (Wang et al., 2025), researchers looked at ETS exposure among children using cotinine levels in blood. Cotinine is a metabolic byproduct of nicotine, so if you find it in the bloodstream of someone who doesn't smoke (for example, in a six-year-old), then it is a marker that they have been exposed to ETS. What the researchers found was that those children in the lowest income bracket had the highest levels of cotinine in their blood. This secondhand smoke exposure among low SES children has been consistently shown, and it is a bit disheartening to see that it is still the case in 2025 (which also happens to be the year in which *The Running Man* takes place).

We know that those of lower SES are more likely to start smoking, and less likely to quit, and they are more likely to be exposed to secondhand smoke when they are young. Back to *The Running Man*, you can see this pattern playing out – we have Ben and Bradley smoking, and we have their young daughter and sister being exposed. Unfortunately for Cathy and Cassie, we can add this to their ecological exposure at the microsystems (and mesosystem if you take SES into account) level. For Cathy, this has probably played a role in her pneumonia – in one recent meta-analysis of children under the age of 5, there was a 2.15 times higher chance of getting pneumonia if you were exposed to secondhand smoke compared to no exposure (Riestiyowati et al., 2020). As for Cassie and her lung cancer, a recent meta-analysis showed that secondhand smoke exposure in the home led to a 20% increase in lung cancer diagnosis (Possenti et al., 2024).

Exosystem Level

On the exosystem level, we have local industry, which is causing a significant "miasma"-like atmosphere in both Co-Op City and Boston (Koch, 2005). The air quality in these areas is so bad that the local governments have stopped publishing the air-pollution counts, in hopes that the people will just "forget." The Free-Vee's help play into this, as they spew an aggressive amount of information regarding climate and public health. This makes it hard to get the correct information, and the correct protective gear, to avoid the harmful effects of the pollution.

Research consistently shows that it is the low SES neighborhoods that are exposed to air with higher concentrations of pollutants (Hajat et al., 2015). The pollution is so bad that the body's natural defenses that I talked about earlier cannot filter out what is being pumped into the air, so in Co-Op City and other places, nose filters are required. Of course, the ones that the people in the polluted areas can afford aren't effective, and the ones that are effective cost thousands of new dollars and are only available to those within the highest ranks of SES. This is how you end up with an 18-month-old with a deadly case of pneumonia and a five-year-old with metastasizing lung cancer.

Macrosystem Level

On the macrosystem level, reflecting the impact of the ideas of the larger government structures on health, we have several factors at play. First, we have some government policies that are meant to reduce the health literacy of the populace, so that they are unaware of the health dangers that they face. One congressional law in this dystopian government that attempts to limit knowledge is the policy regarding library cards. Low SES populations are not allowed to get library cards and use the public library. In order to get a library card, an individual must show that they have a guaranteed yearly income of $5,000 new dollars. When the government only provides benefits of $1,040 old dollars a year – the health-improvement knowledge waiting to be discovered at your local library is well out of your reach.

Bradley and The Stabbers are crafty though – they pick-pocket a library card, get themselves a respectful looking suit, and take their turns heading to the local library. It is here that they learn about the high rates of pollution they are being exposed to and the ineffectiveness of the nose filters they have been provided. With what they learn from the library books, they are able to make their own nose filters, as well as their own air-pollution counters.

One last note on the macrosystem level has to do with unemployment. Unemployment is playing a huge role here for both Cathy and Cassie. The unemployment of their families means that they cannot afford the nutritional food that they need to stay healthy to begin with, and they cannot afford the appropriate healthcare needed now that they are sick. The unemployment that their families face has a lot to do with larger systems infrastructure. Whether it was due to race, financial situations, or other factors beyond their control, the Richardses and the Throckmortons did not have high levels of education – having had to get out in the real world earlier in life. This has made it so that they are only qualified for certain types of jobs – and unfortunately for all involved – their low educational status means they are qualified for dangerous and low-paying work. This has been the plight of Ben Richards – who has had to work in several of the industries that are large polluters and have exposed him to even more chemical and radiological risk than the general public. Many of the people of this dystopian world need to decide between their lives and money. While Ben had been consistently choosing his life (and fertility) over money, Cathy's illness put him over the edge. By becoming a contestant on "The Running Man", he has put his life on the line.

Individual Factor with Impacts across Levels – Race

There have been centuries of racial segregation throughout our country, and the policies and procedures around housing have made racial differences in neighborhood makeup distinct and profound. This includes an uneven distribution of pollution exposure between low social position White neighborhoods and low social position Black neighborhoods – with the Black neighborhood experiencing more pollution than their White counterparts (Clougherty et al., 2022). If this tracks within *The Running Man*, it is safe to assume that Cathy's Co-Op City neighborhood, while still exposed to pollution, was exposed to less of it than Cassie's. This would explain the difference in the severity of their illness – a treatable infectious disease versus metastasized lung cancer.

Another reason for Cassie's more serious diagnosis is due to racial disparities in cancer diagnoses in general. In a recent review article, Zavala and colleagues (2021) found that there are still striking cancer disparities among minority groups in the Unites States, with Black populations seeing high morbidity and mortality rates across a wide range of cancer types (Zavala et al., 2021). Unfortunately, this hasn't changed much since Ward et al. found similar racial differences in 2004.

One proposed mechanism by which minority status "gets under the skin" to affect these health outcomes is the Minority Stress Model (Meyer, 2003). While first developed to explain mental health disparities in sexual minorities, the model has been widely adapted to explain the minority specific stressors encountered by many minority populations. The first thing to understand about the model is that minority stress is different from other types of stress in that it stems from the prejudice and stigma that is placed upon the person due to their minority group status. Stress could include external stressors, such as being exposed to discrimination, violence, microaggressions, and the like. Internally, the individual may internalize the stigma and stereotypes of their minority group, and they may spend energy concealing or separating themselves from their minority status.

These stressors do not just come and go; they are usually chronically experienced by the individual, which creates a constant stress environment that wears away at bodily systems. For example, minority stress has been found to be associated with overall physical health, sleep, and immune and cardiovascular system outcomes (Flentje et al., 2025). Interestingly enough, one of the factors that has been found to have a big impact on minority stress is vigilance – the same factor we talked about with Bill Hodges and his role in law enforcement. The level of vigilance that comes with being a Black person in the United States places a staggering toll on one's health. Race-related vigilance levels in Black US populations have shown to be related to sleep difficulties (Hicken et al., 2013), obesity (Powell et al., 2016), depressive symptoms (Watson-Singleton et al., 2019), and inflammation as measured by levels of C-reactive protein (Davis et al., 2025).

Now you may be saying that Cassie was a bit too young to experience these types of racial experiences, or at least young enough that they would not have impacted her health. I disagree. Her entire family was feeling the effects of minority stress, including vigilance effects, and I am sure their stress had impacts on her. I also think that five is young enough to start understanding the stigma and violence directed at you because of your race – especially in such a dystopian environment as we have here. This, combined with all of the other ecological factors I have discussed here, created a perfect storm for Cassie, which resulted in her devastating illness.

Conclusion

As I stated in the beginning, Stephen King, as Richard Bachman, really knows how to deliver a devastating blow when uncovering the evils of society. *The Running Man* is the perfect example – it is hard to leave the book without thinking about our own societal ills, and how so much of the book may be rooted in reality. Quite a departure from the King horrors we are used to.

The Running Man

Novel: King, S. [as Bachman, R.]. (1982). *The Running Man*. Signet Books.

Audiobook: King, S. [as Bachman, R.]. (1982). *The Running Man* (F. Muller, Narr.) [Audiobook]. Penguin Random House Audio. https://www.penguinrandomhouseaudio.com

Further Explorations

1 Bronfenbrenner's model can be applied to many of Stephen King's novels and short stories. Pick one of your favorite characters and analyze their life circumstances and health and wellbeing based on the model. Provide peer-reviewed evidence to back up your analysis.
2 Take a look at the latest article reviewing the Minority Stress Model (Frost & Meyer, 2023). Using their updated model, discuss Ben Richards as a minority (low SES) in this dystopian society. How does this affect his health, his decisions, and his interactions with others in the novel?

Notes

1 Just as a quick note – for most of the other King works discussed in this book, I have provided information on the movie or television adaptation for possible reference. I do not provide this for *The Running Man* – as I have a hard time seeing how Arnold Schwarzenegger's 1987 action film has anything to do with the book. I mean the main character has the same name, and there is a game called "The Running Man," but after that, the similarities are nonexistent. Please do not watch the movie with connecting it to health psychology as a goal. Watch it for classic lines from Ben Richards like "What a hothead!" after he kills a guy with a flame-thrower.
2 Rage is a difficult story to read, exploring a student's downward spiral into violence, which he takes out on his teacher and classmates. As a Bachman story, this really hit on the real-world dystopia we all experience in the United States – the book was linked to several school shootings. Due to this, King made the decision to allow it to go out of print, and he has no desire to let it go back into circulation.

Bibliography

Berberian, A. G., Gonzalez, D. J., & Cushing, L. J. (2022). Racial disparities in climate change-related health effects in the United States. *Current Environmental Health Reports*, *9*(3), 451–464. https://doi.org/10.1007/s40572-022-00360-w

Braveman, P. (2006). Health disparities and health equity: Concepts and measurement. *Annual Review of Public Health*, *27*(1), 167–194. https://doi.org/10.1146/annurev.publhealth.27.021405.102103

Bronfenbrenner, U. (1977). Toward an experimental ecology of human development. *American Psychologist*, *32*(7), 513. https://doi.org/10.1037/0003-066X.32.7.513

Centers for Disease Control and Prevention. (2025, June 2). *U.S. Cancer Statistics: Lung Cancer Stat Bite*. https://www.cdc.gov/united-states-cancer-statistics/publications/lung-cancer-stat-bite.html

Clougherty, J. E., Humphrey, J. L., Kinnee, E. J., Remigio, R., & Sheffield, P. E. (2022). What is "socioeconomic position (SEP)," and how might it modify air pollution-health associations? Cohering findings, identifying challenges, and disentangling effects of SEP and race in US City settings. *Current Environmental Health Reports*, *9*(3), 355–365. https://doi.org/10.1007/s40572-022-00359-3

Davis, K. M., Knauft, K., Petriello, M., Jiang, Y., & Zilioli, S. (2025). Vigilance and systemic inflammation among middle-aged to older urban African American adults. *Biopsychosocial Science and Medicine*, *87*(5), 316–321. /

Flentje, A., Sunder, G., & Tebbe, E. (2025). Minority stress in relation to biological outcomes among sexual and gender minority people: A systematic review and update.

Journal of Behavioral Medicine, 48(1), 22–42. https://doi.org/10.1007/s10865-024-00539-6

Frost, D. M., & Meyer, I. H. (2023). Minority stress theory: Application, critique, and continued relevance. *Current Opinion in Psychology, 51*, 101579. https://doi.org/10.1016/j.copsyc.2023.101579

Hajat, A., Hsia, C., & O'Neill, M. S. (2015). Socioeconomic disparities and air pollution exposure: A global review. *Current Environmental Health Reports, 2*(4), 440–450. https://doi.org/10.1007/s40572-015-0069-5

Heitner, R., Rogers, M., Chambers, B., Pinotti, R., Silvers, A., Meier, D. E., ... & Johnson, K. S. (2023). The experience of black patients with serious illness in the United States: A scoping review. *Journal of Pain and Symptom Management, 66*(4), e501–e511. https://doi.org/10.1016/j.jpainsymman.2023.07.002

Hicken, M. T., Lee, H., Ailshire, J., Burgard, S. A., & Williams, D. R. (2013). Every shut eye, ain't sleep: The role of racism-related vigilance in racial/ethnic disparities in sleep difficulty. *Race and social problems, 5*(2), 100–112. https://doi.org/10.1007/s12552-013-9095-9

Hiscock, R., Bauld, L., Amos, A., Fidler, J. A., & Munafò, M. (2012). Socioeconomic status and smoking: A review. *Annals of the New York Academy of Sciences, 1248*(1), 107–123. https://doi.org/10.1111/j.1749-6632.2011.06202.x

King, S. (2012). *The Running Man*. Random House. https://www.amazon.com/dp/B0078XGJXO

Koch, T. (2005). Mapping the miasma: Air, health, and place in early medical mapping. *Cartographic Perspectives*, 52, 4–27.

Meyer, I. H. (2003). Prejudice, social stress, and mental health in lesbian, gay, and bisexual populations: Conceptual issues and research evidence. *Psychological Bulletin, 129*(5), 674.

Possenti, I., Romelli, M., Carreras, G., Biffi, A., Bagnardi, V., Specchia, C., ... & Lugo, A. (2024). Association between second-hand smoke exposure and lung cancer risk in never-smokers: A systematic review and meta-analysis. *European Respiratory Review, 33*(174), 240077. https://doi.org/10.1183/16000617.0077-2024

Powell, L. R., Jesdale, W. M., & Lemon, S. C. (2016). On edge: The impact of race-related vigilance on obesity status in African–Americans. *Obesity Science & Practice, 2*(2), 136–143. https://doi.org/10.1002/osp4.42

Reifsnider, E., Gallagher, M., & Forgione, B. (2005). Using ecological models in research on health disparities. *Journal of Professional Nursing, 21*(4), 216–222. https://doi.org/10.1016/j.profnurs.2005.05.006

Riestiyowati, M. A., Rahardjo, S. S., & Murti, B. (2020). A meta-analysis of the effects of secondhand smoke exposure toward the incidence of pneumonia in children under five. *Journal of Epidemiology and Public Health, 5*(4), 410–419. https://doi.org/10.26911/jepublichealth.2020.05.04.03

Vaughn, V. M., Dickson, R. P., Horowitz, J. K., & Flanders, S. A. (2024). Community-acquired pneumonia: A review. *JAMA, 332*(15), 1282–1295. https://doi.org/10.1001/jama.2024.14796

Wang, J., Ma, J., Hu, T., Ye, Y., Zhao, Y., Abulikemu, S., ... & Peng, Y. (2025). Trends of cotinine and secondhand smoke exposure rates in children and adolescent aged 6–19 years: Impact of race and socioeconomic factors over two decades. *Addictive Behaviors*, (170), 108413. https://doi.org/10.1016/j.addbeh.2025.108413

Ward, E., Jemal, A., Cokkinides, V., Singh, G. K., Cardinez, C., Ghafoor, A., & Thun, M. (2004). Cancer disparities by race/ethnicity and socioeconomic status. *CA: A Cancer Journal for Clinicians, 54*(2), 78–93.

Watson-Singleton, N. N., Hill, L. K., & Case, A. D. (2019). Past discrimination, race-related vigilance, and depressive symptoms: The moderating role of mindfulness. *Mindfulness*, *10*(9), 1768–1778. https://doi.org/10.1007/s12671-019-01143-5

Zavala, V. A., Bracci, P. M., Carethers, J. M., Carvajal-Carmona, L., Coggins, N. B., Cruz-Correa, M. R., … & Fejerman, L. (2021). Cancer health disparities in racial/ethnic minorities in the United States. *British Journal of Cancer*, *124*(2), 315–332. https://doi.org/10.1038/s41416-020-01038-6

7 ACEs and *The Body*

Early Life Experiences and Health

You're ACEs Gordie!

When asked what is one of their favorite movies of all time, countless people (my husband included) will list Rob Reiner's 1986 classic *Stand By Me*. Many people are surprised to hear that this is a film adaptation of a Stephen King novella called *The Body* (Another Stephen King adaptation that often makes it on people's favorite movie list is *The Shawshank Redemption*, again, to many people's surprise. King is not just horror!). While this chapter focuses on *The Body* novella (see Box 7.1 for summary), the movie is quite amazing, and it is incorporated into the assignment questions at the end – so movie fans have no fear!

Box 7.1 ***The Body***

The Body takes place in 1960s Castle Rock (home of Alan Pangborn from *The Dark Half*, see Chapter 3). It revolves around a summer adventure embarked upon by four 12-year-old friends: Chris Chambers, Teddy Duchamp, Gordie Lachance, and Vern Tessio. Following the news of a missing boy, the friends overhear the local town bullies discussing a body that they found by the train tracks. The bullies have opted not to report the body, since they were participating in some illegal doings when it was discovered. The boys decide that they will go and find the body themselves – out of curiosity and the want to become famous.

⚠ **[Spoiler Alert]** The four set out to follow the train tracks, armed with a gun that Chris Chambers stole from his dad. Hijinks ensue, as the boys are attacked at the town dump by the legendary Chopper (the second most legendary dog in town, after Cujo), have a close call with the train on a bridge, and become food for a pond full of leeches. Eventually, they do reach the body, but with unfortunate timing. The town bullies, led by Ace Merrril, have also returned to the body. The boys and bullies tussle over who gets to claim the body, and the fight comes to a halt when Chris pulls the gun on Ace.

DOI: 10.4324/9781003495994-7

The gun drives the bullies away, and the boys, feeling overwhelmed by their "adventure," return home.

As they leave, the bullies vow to make the boys pay. That they do – with all four boys being beaten by Ace and company toward the end of the story. We also see how the boys, despite having such a bonding experience, drift apart, and go their separate ways. The story, which is being told by Gordie Lachance, who has become a famous author, describes the ultimate fate of each boy, as well as Ace Merrill.

An Introduction to Adverse Childhood Experiences

What makes *The Body* interesting from a health psychology standpoint is the hardships that each boy faces – not just on their journey down the railroad tracks, but their journey through childhood. Each of the four friends has had their fair share of adverse childhood experiences (ACEs). While this story takes place in the 1960s, it wasn't until the 1990s that ACEs started to be explored as a predictor of health and wellbeing.

The original ACEs study (Felitti et al., 1998) looked at almost 10,000 US adults who were examined at Kaiser Permanente's San Diego Health Appraisal Clinic. After the participants had received a full physical examination at the clinic, they were sent a questionnaire that asked them a wide range of questions regarding what their life was like growing up. In total, seven abuse and dysfunction categories were assessed, and participants were asked to state whether they had occurred in the first 18 years or their lives. The questions were as follows:

1. **Abuse: Psychological**
   - Did a parent or other adult in the household:
     - Swear at, insult, or put you down?
     - Act in a way that made you feel afraid that you would be physically hurt?
2. **Abuse: Physical**
   - Did a parent or other adult in the household:
     - Push, grab, shove, or slap you?
     - Hit you so hard that you had marks or were injured?
3. **Abuse: Sexual**
   - Did an adult or person at least five years older ever:
     - Touch or fondle you in a sexual way?
     - Have you touch their body in a sexual way?
     - Attempt oral, anal, or vaginal intercourse with you?
     - Actually have oral, anal, or vaginal intercourse with you?

4 **Household Dysfunction: Substance Abuse**

- Did you live with anyone who was a problem drinker or alcoholic?
- Did you live with anyone who used street drugs?

5 **Household Dysfunction: Mental Illness**

- Was a household member depressed or mentally ill?
- Did a household member attempt suicide?

6 **Household Dysfunction: Mother treated Violently**

- Was your mother (or stepmother):
  - Pushed, grabbed, slapped, or had something thrown at her?
  - Kicked, bitten, hit with a fist, or hit with something hard?
  - Ever repeatedly hit for at least a few minutes?
  - Every threatened with, or hurt by, a knife or gun?

7 **Household Dysfunction: Criminal Behavior**

- Did a household member go to prison?

If participants answered with a sometimes, often, or very often, or a "yes" for each category, they were given 1 point. Thus, people's ACEs score could range from 0 to 7, with 0 being no exposure to ACEs, and 7 being exposure to all of the ACEs. About 52% of the participants in the study endorsed having at least one of these experiences, and about 6% reported having four or more.

The researchers then looked at how people scored on the ACEs questionnaire in terms of their current health and wellbeing. First, they looked at ten risk factors that have been shown to impact morbidity and mortality (remember the epidemiologists bathtub!). These were: smoking, severe obesity, physical inactivity, depressed mood, suicide attempts, alcohol abuse, drug abuse, parental drug abuse, number of sexual partners, and history of sexually transmitted disease. The researcher also looked at specific diseases within the participants, such as ischemic heart disease, cancer, stroke, chronic obstructive pulmonary disease, diabetes, hepatitis, and skeletal fractures. Lastly, they simply asked participants whether they felt they were physically healthy.

What they found may have been well understood by many, but for the first time was demonstrated by a wealth of data – experiencing ACEs was not good for your health and health behaviors as an adult. Let's look at a few examples:

Being a current smoker:

- Scoring a 2 on the ACEs questionnaire was associated with a 50% higher chance of being a current smoker than scoring a 0
- Scoring a 3 on the ACEs questionnaire was associated with a 100% higher chance of being a current smoker than scoring a 0
- Scoring a 4 or higher was associated with a 120% increase.

Considers self an alcoholic:

- Scoring a 1 was associated with a 100% increase in the chance of labeling oneself an alcoholic
- Scoring a 2 was associated with a 200% increase in the chance of labeling oneself as an alcoholic
- Scoring a 3 was associated with a 390% increase in the chance of labeling oneself as an alcoholic
- Scoring a 4 or more was associated with a 640% increase in the chance of labeling oneself as an alcoholic.

Has ischemic heart disease (coronary heart disease):

- Those who scored a 3 on the ACEs questionnaire had a 40% higher chance of having ischemic heart disease than those who scored a 0.
- Those who scored a 4 or higher on the ACEs questionnaire had a 120% higher chance of having ischemic heart disease than those who scored 0

Has any cancer:

- Those who scored a 4 or higher on the ACEs questionnaire had a 90% higher chance of having cancer than those who scored a 0.

These strong associations were seen for most of the risk factors and diseases they looked at. These associations were also adjusted for age, gender, race, and education. Needless to say, these findings were very impactful when they were first published, and they put ACEs on the radar of health providers everywhere. These findings have been replicated numerous times (e.g. Bellis et al., 2019; Bhutta et al., 2023; Hughes et al., 2017), and it is not surprising to see ACEs questionnaires given as part of physical and mental health assessments throughout the world.

So how does this bode for our four favorite tween adventurers in Castle Rock? It is not good. See Table 7.1 for how I would score Chris, Teddy, Gordie, and Vern on the original ACEs criteria.

So how does this work? How do these scores "get under the skin" to impact adult health, at least in terms of the gang from *The Body*? Well, let's look at the first obvious one, smoking (for more details on this health-compromising behavior, see Chapter 10). In *The Body*, we have a group of 11–12-year-old boys who smoke cigarettes on a regular basis. They meet up at a treehouse, playing cards and smoking cigarettes – so many in fact that the treehouse is filled with ashtrays. Most of them score a two or higher on the original questionnaire, which would increase their risk of being a smoker by 50%. In the case of Chris Chambers, his risk is increased by 120% compared to someone with no ACEs.[1]

For all that these four go through, I personally feel that their ACEs scores are low and not reflective of all the adverse events they experience. And this was even pointed out in the original ACEs study, where they suggest that future

Table 7.1 ACEs Scored for the Main Protagonist of *The Body*

Character	*Original 7-Items ACEs Questionnaire*	
	Question Endorsed	*Point*
Chris Chambers	Psychological abuse	1
	Physical abuse	1
	Substance abuse	1
	Criminal household behavior	1
	Total ACEs score	4
Teddy Duchamp	Physical abuse	1
	Mental illness	1
	Total ACEs score	2
Gordie Lachance	Mental illness (depression)	1
	Total ACEs score	1
Vern Tessio	Psychological abuse	1
	Physical abuse	1
	Total ACEs score	2

researchers should consider casting an even wider net when it comes to potential ACEs. Since the original study was published in 1998, a plethora of questionnaires have been developed that assess additional ACEs, most notably the loss of a parent through death, divorce, and abandonments, and the inclusion of a negligence category.

Most recently, a study by D'Arcy-Bewick and colleagues (2023) created a more comprehensive list of 20 ACEs based on a multitude of questionnaires that were asked in the MIDUS study – a large longitudinal cohort study of mid-life adults in the United States. Participants could score between 0 and 20. The categories and 20 questions included:

Physical Abuse

- How often did one of the above push, grab, or shove you
- How often did the above slap you
- How often did one of the above throw something at you
- How often did one of the above kick, bite, or hit you with a fist
- How often did one of the above beat you
- How often did one of the above choke you
- How often did one of the above burn or scald you

Emotional Abuse

- How frequently did mother, father, sibling, or other insult or swear at you
- How often did one of the above sulk or refuse to talk to you
- How often did one of the above say or do something spiteful
- How often did one of the above threaten to hit you
- How often did one of the above smash or kick something in anger

Disadvantaged Socioeconomic Status (SES)
- Family receipt of welfare or assistance for children for six months or longer
- Head of household has less than a college education
- Self-report of being worse off than other families

Poor Physical Health at Age 16

Poor Mental Health at Age 16

Adverse Family Structure
- Parents divorced
- Lack of father figure in household
- Death of parent

When we look at the boys from this lens, I think their scores make a bit more sense. Chris jumps to around 13, and Teddy gets around an eight. One important addition here is that of SES. Take a look at Chapter 6 for more information on why socioeconomic factors might be particularly detrimental to someone's health. Before we start going into too many more particulars about the health outcomes, let's take a look at each character and see (1) how they got the scores they did and the (2) how that score may be getting "under their skin" to impact their health – and unfortunately – their mortality.

Teddy Duchamp – The Risk Taker

We will start with Teddy Duchamp, who seems to have the clearest connection between what is going on in his home life and what may be happening to him on a biopsychosocial level. Teddy earns his ACEs score mostly due to his father – a World War 2 vet who has been suffering from significant PTSD since he "stormed the beach at Normandy." Teddy's dad, Norman Duchamp, is Section 8,[2] which in the 1960s means he received a military discharge, and is currently hospitalized for mental health reasons stemming from his service. What finally placed Norman in Togus (the VA hospital) was an incident that occurred when Teddy was eight and he broke a plate. Norman was so incensed by this that he grabbed Teddy and held his head down on the hot burner plate of the stove in the kitchen. He first seared one side of Teddy's face (mostly getting the ear), lifted him up, and then seared the other. The police and ambulance were called after a neighbor heard Teddy's painful screams, and Norman was seen toting his gun around, grumbling about snipers around every corner.

After this incident, Norman was permanently removed from the Duchamps' home. In order to make ends meet, his mother started renting out rooms in the house, in addition to working her job at the shoe factory. The episode with the oven earns Teddy two points on the original ACEs questionnaire (one for physical abuse, and one for mental illness of a family member). This abuse would earn him more points on the ACEs-20 – I think he gets at least three points based on the physical abuse questions.

Stemming from his father's abuse, Teddy lost much of his hearing, and is required to wear hearing aids, as well as thick glasses for his eyesight. For this, he earns another point for the ACEs-20 physical health category. Neither of his parents were college-educated; they probably received government assistance from Norman's time in the service, and chances are they are now on a fixed income. I would suspect that this, along with the renters and long hours at the shoe factory, would lead to a self-report of being "worse off than other families." This gives Teddy three more points on the ACEs-20. Add the fact that his father is no longer with them (+1), Teddy's total ACES-20 score is an eight, and a two on the original scale. I suspect that if we spent a week, or even a day, with Teddy and his family while his dad was still there, this would be higher (and the original study showed that if you have one ACE, your chances of having others increase significantly).

With Teddy, you do not need to wait until adulthood to see how all of this is impacting him physically and mentally. Teddy is described by his friends as the crazy one – and there is no better proof of this than his penchant for "truck-dodging." There is nothing that Teddy likes better than running out in front of the fast-moving trucks on Route 196. He also takes any dares that come his way. Teddy is constantly seeking the rush.

This risk-taking may be a result of "cortisol dampening," or hypocortisolism, that has been hypothesized to occur when someone is exposed to extreme trauma conditions and prolonged stress. Here, we have to go back to the HPA axis and stress response that was discussed in Chapter 1. You can imagine that throughout Teddy's life, he has been subjected to a constant state of threat. Living with a father whose PTSD causes him to see threats everywhere, including his own son, probably led to continuous fight or flight responses from Teddy. As we have learned, the more your body perceives threat, the more it will instigate the HPA-axis response that results in an increased release of cortisol from the adrenal glands.

Research has shown that as a result of this constant HPA-axis activity, especially at a young age, a paradoxical phenomenon happens where you start producing less cortisol. In a recent meta-analysis, Brindle and colleagues (2022) found that ACEs were associated with lower levels of cortisol, as well as less cardiovascular reactivity. In essence, when faced with constant stressors, your body does not produce stress hormones, and it also slows increases in blood pressure and heart rate that normally occur. This, of course, may be advantageous in the short term – if Teddy reacted to every threatening situation he encountered in an extreme biological way, he would not have the time or resources to do much of anything else. The idea here is that after repeated exposures to ACEs, the body will dampen your cortisol response so it won't "get under your skin" at the moment. Instead, it allows you to continue on with the tasks of life, even in the face of constant trauma and stress.

Again, helpful in the short term, but biologically and psychologically, we are going to see some long-term ramifications. This blunted fight or flight response may be causing Teddy to go out and seek extreme situations to get that biological reaction. One interesting study looked at this hypothesis in vervet monkeys (Laudenslager et al., 2011). In this paradigm, they will put a new and potentially threatening object (snake, tarantula) within reach of the monkeys. They then measure how quickly the monkeys will approach the object and how many times they will return to it in a 30-minute session. The researchers also collected average cortisol levels in the monkeys over time by using cortisol markers in their hair. What they found was that the monkeys who had the lowest cortisol levels approached the threatening object the quickest and repeatedly returned to it to investigate. In essence, the monkeys with the lowest cortisol levels were the most likely to seek out and interact with a potentially risky object.

It is a bit harder to study this in humans, as exposing them to truly threatening or risky situations would never get past an ethics review board. However, one thing that can be seen as scary and threatening by most people is public speaking. One study (Ouellet-Morin et al., 2011), which comes from a twin cohort like we discussed in Chapter 3,[3] looked at 190 12-year-olds who were exposed to an adapted Trier Social Stress Test (Kirschbaum et al., 1993). In this task, the children were interviewed by a research assistant, while also being videotaped. They were first asked to do a difficult addition task, in which they were told to make as few mistakes as possible, because they were in competition with their twin to win a prize. They were then asked to do the public speaking task, which required them to speak for five minutes straight about an unpleasant experience they had at school – all while a judge and interviewer watched. This is one of the most threatening situations you can put someone in ethically.

The researchers also assessed the children's exposure to maltreatment in the home, as well as frequent bullying. When they compared the children who had high rates of maltreatment/bullying to those children with low rates, they found that the maltreated/bullied children had significantly lower cortisol response to the stressor. The maltreated/bullied children barely registered a cortisol response.

All this is to say that Teddy's extreme adverse life events have probably caused some significant developmental changes in how his stress response works. This change may make him more likely to take the risks he does. What might this mean for the adult Teddy? He could be in store for more adult related risk behaviors – for example, pathological gamblers show similar hypocortisolism (Paris et al., 2010). In another study that looked at over 45,000 adults, having high ACEs scores was indicative of risky binge drinking, heavy drinking, smoking, and risky sexual behavior (Campbell et al., 2016).

⚠ **[Spoiler Alert]** Unfortunately, we know how this story ends for Teddy. Despite struggles in middle and high school, he does graduate, and he gets a job with Castle Rock Public Works. But those risky behaviors caught up to him – at 23, he was driving around in his Chevy Bel Air with a bunch of friends, drinking and smoking marijuana, when he crashed into a utility pole, killing them all.

Chris Chambers – The Best Friend

Out of the four boys, Chris Chambers has the most ACEs he will have to overcome. His father is an alcoholic who beats him – sometimes so badly he can't attend school, or he requires an overnight stay in the hospital. In the original ACEs study, he would get two points for this – one for substance abuse and household dysfunction and one for the physical abuse. In the ACEs-20, based on the different types of physical abuse suffered, he would get around six points.

His dad is also a "mean" drunk, who verbally berates his son, among various other emotional manipulations. He would get one point for the original ACEs here, and my guess is around four points for the emotional abuse section of the ACEs-20. We don't have too much information on his mother, or the role she plays within the family dynamic of violence, so we can't say much about mother-based family dysfunction for the original ACEs. We do have information about the Chambers' SES for the ACEs-20. He would likely receive a three here. The Chamberses live in a three-room shack that has no indoor plumbing and little protection from the elements due to a number of broken windows, his dad is uneducated and unemployed and receives welfare sporadically. They are definitely worse off than any other families in Castle Rock – a fact that everyone seems to recognize.

Lastly, the Chambers family is often afoul of the law. His brother Frank spent quite some time in prison for assault and rape, and his other brother "Eyeball" is on the juvenile delinquent track. This gives him an additional point for the original ACEs score. This leaves him with a total score of four in the original ACEs study (four and above is usually considered the highest exposure category) and a 13 in the ACEs-20 (equally high). As Gordie laments "Chris came from a bad family, all right, and everyone thought he would turn out bad...including Chris" (King, 2017, p.19).

In the statement above lies a clue to the negative outcomes Chris is experiencing due to his high adverse events exposure. Chris is an amazing friend – he truly believes in Gordie, and Gordie's ability to become an amazing writer. What he doesn't believe in is himself. He has so much energy and support to give his friend – but nothing to give himself. We can categorize this as internalized negative beliefs, learned hopelessness, and a lack of self-efficacy. That is a lot of psychological jargon, so let's break it down.

Internalized negative beliefs refer to the phenomena that occurs when someone is repeatedly told something about themselves. For Chris, he received a lot of messages from people around him, especially his father – that he was worthless, stupid, wouldn't amount to anything – the list goes on and on. The whole town thinks that the Chambers family is good-for-nothing – Chris included. This extends to the teachers and administrators at school. One striking example is the case of the missing milk money. When the milk money goes missing at school, no one even asks – it is just assumed that Chris took it. Assumed guilty, he was given three days' detention. It never once occurred to him to defend himself – he knows everyone viewed him as a hopeless screw-up. He has heard this so many times, he now believes it himself.

However, what actually happened was he had taken the milk money but then returned it to the teacher. The teacher never returned it to the school, using it to buy a new skirt instead. Chris understands that there is no way to tell the administrators this – they would never believe him. The teacher knew this, so it was the perfect crime in a sense. Thinking about this brings tears to the normally stoic boy's eyes. He has learned that no matter what he does, he can't change his circumstances, or how he is viewed by the people around him. This is what we call learned helplessness (Seligman & Maier, 1967).

The result of Chris' internalized negative beliefs about himself and his learned helplessness is he has low levels of self-efficacy. Self-efficacy is an important concept that was developed by Albert Bandura in 1977 to explain aspects of behavior change (we will talk about it in this context in Chapter 10). Bandura proposed that self-efficacy was your own belief in your capabilities – your understanding of your ability to do what needs to be done to manage situations and challenges facing you. Bandura stated that there were some key elements to self-efficacy, and unfortunately Chris has significant deficits in each. First, you must have examples of when you successfully did something. Due to his internalized negative beliefs, it is hard to see that he would recognize life success (Gordie tries to convince him of his intelligence, to no avail). You also need to learn what success looks like through vicarious experience. Knowing the Chambers family, he has little in the role model department. Next, you need verbal encouragement from others, and we know he is getting the exact opposite. Lastly, you need to have a positive mood/outlook, and reduced stress levels. All of these requirements demonstrate why Chris is low on self-efficacy.

Studies repeatedly show that childhood maltreatment and adversity impact all of the above psychological outcomes (see Li et al., 2020 for review). These then can lead to numerous deleterious health and wellbeing outcomes, such as increased depression (Li et al., 2020; Pryce et al., 2011), altered immune function (Caserta et al., 2011; Hladek et al., 2020), and risky health behaviors (Schwarzer & Fuchs, 1995; Schwarzer & Luszczynska, 2006).

⚠ **[Spoiler Alert]** The outlook for Chris isn't good. Yet, with the unwavering support of Gordie, he began to take more difficult courses and succeeded. Despite the naysaying of almost everyone around him, he was accepted to the University of Maine at Portland, pre-law. Unfortunately, his high ACEs score caught up with him. We have seen that those with the highest ACEs scores die on average 20 years earlier than those with no ACEs. Chris was not even given that much time. At age 24, he is fatally stabbed while trying to break up a fight at a Portland chicken restaurant.

Gordie Lachance – Neglected but Resilient

Next up is Gordie Lachance, who on the surface seems to be doing much better than his counterparts in the ACEs department – after all, his parents aren't abusive, right? While we don't know what Gordie's parents do (or did, his dad is retired), he seems a bit better off financially than his friends. In this, he doesn't earn any SES points in the ACEs-20. We do know that he has just lost his older brother Denny in an accident that occurred during Army basic training. There was a significant age difference between Gordie and Denny, so how close they were or weren't is something Gordie grapples with, but his parents are devastated. Denny was their first, and in some respects, only child – their golden boy, who they set all their hopes on, mostly neglecting Gordie. His parents' grief and depression following Denny's death is why Gordie gets a one on the original ACEs score.

While Gordie had always played second fiddle to Denny, after his death, this neglect becomes even more acute. While negligence is not listed on either the original

ACEs or the ACEs-20, it is considered a form of maltreatment. In some sense, what Gordie's parents are doing would be called unintentional child neglect – I don't think they have any idea the toll their lack of care and concern has placed on Gordie.

In one study, it was shown that children were twice as likely to experience unintentional neglect when a parent is depressed (Friedman & Billick, 2015). We actually have a lot of data regarding the short- and long-term health outcomes of such neglect in childhood. This is because neglect is the most common form of childhood maltreatment in the United States (Daley et al., 2025). Some health characteristics of neglected children include obesity, nutritional deficiencies, and untreated illnesses and injuries (Leeb et al., 2011). As adults, neglected children have an increased risk of drug use, depressive and anxiety disorders, suicidal behavior, suicide attempt, suicidal ideation, and sexually transmitted diseases (Norman et al., 2012). Thus, even though he scores only a one on the original ACEs questions, and a zero on the ACEs-20, he is still at considerable risk.

Despite all this, Gordie is the only one who is still alive as an adult, and he is a successful writer to boot. One of the reasons for Gordie's success is resiliency – a person's ability to successfully adapt in the face of adversity and significant stressors (Masten & Reed, 2002). In one qualitative systematic review, it was found that when exposed to childhood adversity, those who showed more self-reliance were likely to exhibit more resiliency when they were adults (Leung et al., 2022). Here, the fact that Gordie's parents neglected him, and pretty much left him on his own, may have provided him with the psychological toolbox he needed.

In addition, Gordie had a true champion in his best friend Chris Chambers, who made him see his talent and potential. This helped immensely with what we would call Gordie's "self-system functioning" – which includes a positive self-concept, increased self-esteem, and self-efficacy. The self-system functioning also included the things that make Gordie a good writer – his self-awareness, capacity to reflect, and his motivation and drive to eventually become a great writer. Resiliency researchers recognize that this self-system functioning is important for resiliency in maltreated children (Cicchetti, 2013).

Gordie survives the potential negative impacts of his childhood – lucky for us, as he is the one telling us the story!

Vern Tessio – The Unknown

Vern Tessio is the one in the group we know the least about. We know he has an older brother named Billy, who bullies him and beats him up all the time. While Billy is not technically an adult, I consider him close enough to give Vern a two on the original ACEs scale. I also think this abuse would give him around a seven on the ACEs-20. Most of his adverse experiences relate to his brother, as he seems to have a good relationship with his parents. We also know that his dad works at the mill and owns a 1952 Desota, but other than that, we know little about his SES or the other categories of ACEs.

⚠ **[Spoiler Alert]** There are two things we can say about Vern in relation to his ACEs. One is that we know Vern is overweight, and several review papers have shown that ACEs are significantly associated with childhood obesity (Moriya et al., 2024; Schroeder et al., 2021). The other is that he fell victim to the early mortality that is associated with ACEs – at 18, he died in a house fire during a party.

Conclusion

This was a rough chapter to write, as all of these boys deserved better than what life handed them, and three of them deserved more time on this earth than what they were given. I have tried to lighten the mood a bit with the inclusion of Box 7.2, an analysis of the story Gordie tells the others around the campfire. Despite this, it is hard to talk about ACEs without feeling the enormous weight of all we can't protect children from, and how those traumas of childhood continue haunting them throughout their lives. While this isn't a book about clinical psychology, if I ever write one, I will make sure to include all the information about treatments and interventions for lessening the impact of ACEs – there is hope!

Box 7.2 The Revenge of Lard Ass Hogan

I don't think we can talk about *The Body* without discussing the trials and tribulations of Davie Hogan – and lucky for us, I can make a connection between his story and health psychology!

In a very "meta" turn, while older Gordie is telling the story of the trip to find the dead body, younger Gordie, within that story, tells a story around the campfire about Davie "Lard Ass" Hogan, who joins a pie-eating contest during his town's Pioneer Days. The twist of the story is that Davie doesn't join the contest to win, he joins the contest to get revenge on all of the town folks who take so much joy in mocking his weight and calling him names.

Before the pie-eating contest begins, Davie chugs down a bottle of castor oil. For those of you who aren't familiar, castor oil is a type of vegetable oil that is used as a purgative – it will start the "purging" of waste from your body. This is exactly what Davie is hoping for.

While he is expertly taking down his competitors at the pie-eating contest, his stomach begins to make devious noises, and his gag reflex is set into full gear. Well into his fifth pie, Davie can no longer hold back, and projectile vomit (blueberry in nature) meets its target by hitting his competitor. What happens next is that Pioneer Days turns into an absolute Barfarama (credit to Wil Wheaton in *Stand By Me*). The competitors start vomiting, as do the judges, the townspeople, everyone – just as Davie had hoped.

In a way, this is what we might call a Mass Psychogenic Illness – when a group of people all develop the same symptoms, or similar symptoms. without any shared organic etiology (cause). No one else at Pioneer Days ate five blueberry pies in quick succession, or downed a bottle of castor oil – so why are they all throwing up? There may be several biopsychosocial mechanisms at work here:

Mirror Neurons

Mirror neurons are specialized neurons in the brain that activate similar to us performing a task when we are actually just watching someone else do the task. To explain this better, let me tell you the story of how mirror neurons were discovered. Basically, there was a monkey in a lab, and its brain was measured for electrical activity. When the monkey reached for something, say a banana, then, a certain set of neurons would fire. Amazingly enough, when the monkey saw the experimenter reach for a banana, the same neurons would fire. Thus, it was discovered that certain neurons will fire when you are doing an action and when you watch someone else doing the action (Gallese et al., 1996).

Researchers theorize that these neurons may be the source of empathy, or how we put ourselves into other people's emotions. Mirror neurons may fire when you see someone disgusted to the point of vomiting, and then you do so yourself (Rizzolatti and Caruana, 2017; Wicker et al., 2003). It could be that mirror neurons were to blame for Pioneer Days Barfarama.

Survival of the Most Disgusted?

Our brain and body may be endowed with a gag reflex that is particularly sensitive to seeing others throwing up, in an effort to prevent ourselves from being poisoned by contaminated food and being exposed to other pathogens (Oaten et al., 2009).

This may be one of the key connections between our mind and our body. When you feel the overwhelming emotion of disgust, it can initiate a gag reflex, which then can cause you to throw up, thus ridding yourself of the toxin.

Conditioned Response

We will talk about conditioned responses in terms of rats in psychoimmunology (Chapter 8) and in smokers (Chapter 10), but it could also be at play here. If one of the audience members has had a pretty horrible experience with vomiting in the past, just the sights, sounds, and smells associated with someone else throwing up could lead to a conditioned response. We can see this all the time in chemotherapy – a previous neutral stimulus, like the outpatient clinic, or the registration nurse, becomes associated with the nausea of chemotherapy. Once this association occurs, the person can become sick just by looking at the clinic, or the nurse, prior to any chemotherapy treatment (Tomoyasu et al., 1996).

All of these could also play a role in the development of vomiting phobia – called emetophobia. Luckily, emetophobia, as defined by the DSM-5, is fairly rare (Keyes et al., 2018) – so I hope you are all doing alright after reading this box!

The Body

Novella: King, S. (1982). *The Body*. In *Different Seasons*.Viking Press.
Audiobook: King, S. (2016). *The Body* (F. Muller, Narr.). Simon & Schuster Audio. https://www.amazon.com/dp/1508218552
Movie: Reiner, R. (Director). (1986). *Stand By Me* [Film]. Columbia Pictures.

Further Explorations

1 Of course, it is not just the four friends who have the hardships; other characters like Ace Merrill have also had their fair share of ACEs. Fill out additional rows in Table 7.1 for other characters. Justify your inclusions.
2 Take a look at the scores I give the boys for both the original ACEs 7-point scale and the revised 20-point scale. Did I get them right? Why or why not? What scores would you have given them? What scores would they have given themselves – that is, do you think they would have endorsed everything they've experienced if asked to fill out the questionnaire themselves? Why might they answer differently for themselves than how we would answer for them?
3 Watch the movie *Stand By Me* – does it do a good job illustrating the ACEs of each character? Why or why not? Does it give any sense of the negative outcomes of those ACEs might be?
4 What do you think about Vern Tessio – the unknown? What conclusion about his home life and his ACEs score can you extrapolate from what little information about him we are given? How do you think this impacts his health and wellbeing? Why?
5 Thinking about how the emotion of disgust can be "contagious" – what other human emotions and biological functions are contagious? How is it evolutionarily advantageous for us to "catch" these emotions or functions from one another?

Notes

1 In the movie, Chris Chambers, portrayed by River Phoenix, is often seen with a cigarette.
2 Today, in the US, Section 8 refers to vouchers that can be used by low SES individuals and families, as well as seniors and those with disabilities. to help make housing affordable. Section 8 vouchers can be used to pay up to 70% of a qualified individual's rent.
3 This one was the Environmental Risk Longitudinal Twin study, which follows twins that were born in England and Wales in 1994 and 1995.

Bibliography

Bandura, A. (1977). Self-efficacy: Toward a unifying theory of behavioral change. *Psychological Review*, *84*(2), 191–215.

Bellis, M. A., Hughes, K., Ford, K., Rodriguez, G. R., Sethi, D., & Passmore, J. (2019). Life course health consequences and associated annual costs of adverse childhood experiences across Europe and North America: A systematic review and meta-analysis. *The Lancet Public Health*, *4*(10), e517–e528. https://doi.org/10.1016/S2468-2667(19)30145-8

Bhutta, Z. A., Bhavnani, S., Betancourt, T. S., Tomlinson, M., & Patel, V. (2023). Adverse childhood experiences and lifelong health. *Nature Medicine*, *29*(7), 1639–1648. https://doi.org/10.1038/s41591-023-02426-0

Brindle, R. C., Pearson, A., & Ginty, A. T. (2022). Adverse childhood experiences (ACEs) relate to blunted cardiovascular and cortisol reactivity to acute laboratory stress: A systematic review and meta-analysis. *Neuroscience & Biobehavioral Reviews*, *134*, 104530. https://doi.org/10.1016/j.neubiorev.2022.104530

Brown, D. W., Anda, R. F., Tiemeier, H., Felitti, V. J., Edwards, V. J., Croft, J. B., & Giles, W. H. (2009). Adverse childhood experiences and the risk of premature mortality. *American Journal of Preventive Medicine*, *37*(5), 389–396. https://doi.org/10.1016/j.amepre.2009.06.021

Campbell, J. A., Walker, R. J., & Egede, L. E. (2016). Associations between adverse childhood experiences, high-risk behaviors, and morbidity in adulthood. *American Journal of Preventive Medicine*, *50*(3), 344–352. https://doi.org/10.1016/j.amepre.2015.07.022

Caserta, M. T., Wyman, P. A., Wang, H., Moynihan, J., & O'Connor, T. G. (2011). Associations among depression, perceived self-efficacy, and immune function and health in preadolescent children. *Development and Psychopathology*, *23*(4), 1139–1147. https://doi.org/10.1017/S0954579411000526

Cicchetti, D. (2013). Annual research review: Resilient functioning in maltreated children–past, present, and future perspectives. *Journal of Child Psychology and Psychiatry*, *54*(4), 402–422. https://doi.org/10.1111/j.1469-7610.2012.02608.x/

D'Arcy-Bewick, S., Turiano, N., Sutin, A. R., Terracciano, A., & O'Súilleabháin, P. S. (2023). Adverse childhood experiences and all-cause mortality risk in adulthood. *Child Abuse & Neglect*, *144*, 106386. https://doi.org/10.1016/j.chiabu.2023.106386

Daley, S. F., Gonzalez, D., Bethencourt Mirabal, A., & others. (2025). Child abuse and neglect. In StatPearls. StatPearls Publishing. https://www.ncbi.nlm.nih.gov/books/NBK459146/

Felitti, V. J., Anda, R. F., Nordenberg, D., Williamson, D. F., Spitz, A. M., Edwards, V., Koss, M. P., & Marks, J. S. (1998). Relationship of childhood abuse and household dysfunction to many of the leading causes of death in adults: The adverse childhood experiences (ACE) study. *American Journal of Preventive Medicine*, *14*(4), 245–258. https://doi.org/10.1016/s0749-3797(98)00017-8

Friedman, E., & Billick, S. B. (2015). Unintentional child neglect: Literature review and observational study. *Psychiatric Quarterly*, *86*(2), 253–259. https://doi.org/10.1007/s11126-014-9328-0

Gallese, V., Fadiga, L., Fogassi, L., & Rizzolatti, G. (1996). Action recognition in the premotor cortex. *Brain*, *119*(2), 593–609.

Hladek, M., Gill, J., Lai, C., Lorig, K., & Szanton, S. (2020). High coping self-efficacy associated with lower sweat inflammatory cytokines in adults: A pilot study. *Biological Research for Nursing*, *22*(1), 75–81. https://doi.org/10.1177/1099800419870607

Hughes, K., Bellis, M. A., Hardcastle, K. A., Sethi, D., Butchart, A., Mikton, C., … & Dunne, M. P. (2017). The effect of multiple adverse childhood experiences on health: A systematic review and meta-analysis. *The Lancet Public Health, 2*(8), e356–e366. https://doi.org/10.1016/S2468-2667(17)30118-4

Keyes, A., Gilpin, H. R., & Veale, D. (2018). Phenomenology, epidemiology, co-morbidity and treatment of a specific phobia of vomiting: A systematic review of an understudied disorder. *Clinical Psychology Review, 60*, 15–31. https://doi.org/10.1016/j.cpr.2017.12.002

King, S. (2017). *The Body*. Scribner. https://www.amazon.com/dp/B00P42WROG

Kirschbaum, C., Pirke, K. M., & Hellhammer, D. H. (1993). The 'Trier Social Stress Test'–a tool for investigating psychobiological stress responses in a laboratory setting. *Neuropsychobiology, 28*(1–2), 76–81.

Laudenslager, M. L., Jorgensen, M. J., Grzywa, R., & Fairbanks, L. A. (2011). A novelty seeking phenotype is related to chronic hypothalamic-pituitary-adrenal activity reflected by hair cortisol. *Physiology & Behavior, 104*(2), 291–295. https://doi.org/10.1016/j.physbeh.2011.03.003

Leeb, R. T., Lewis, T., & Zolotor, A. J. (2011). A review of physical and mental health consequences of child abuse and neglect and implications for practice. *American Journal of Lifestyle Medicine, 5*(5), 454–468. https://doi.org/10.1177/1559827611410266

Leung, D. Y., Chan, A. C., & Ho, G. W. (2022). Resilience of emerging adults after adverse childhood experiences: A qualitative systematic review. *Trauma, Violence, & Abuse, 23*(1), 163–181. https://doi.org/10.1177/1524838020933865

Li, E. T., Luyten, P., & Midgley, N. (2020). Psychological mediators of the association between childhood emotional abuse and depression: A systematic review. *Frontiers in Psychiatry, 11*, 559213. https://doi.org/10.3389/fpsyt.2020.559213

Masten, A. S., & Reed, M. G. J. (2002). Resilience in development. *Handbook of Positive Psychology, 74*(2), 74–88.

Moriya, R. M., de Oliveira, C. E. C., Reiche, E. M. V., Passini, J. L. L., & Nunes, S. O. V. (2024). Association of adverse childhood experiences and overweight or obesity in adolescents: A systematic review and network analysis. *Obesity Reviews, 25*(11), e13809. https://doi.org/10.1111/obr.13809

Norman, R. E., Byambaa, M., De, R., Butchart, A., Scott, J., & Vos, T. (2012). The long-term health consequences of child physical abuse, emotional abuse, and neglect: A systematic review and meta-analysis. *PLoS Medicine, 9*(11), e1001349. https://doi.org/10.1371/journal.pmed.1001349

Oaten, M., Stevenson, R. J., & Case, T. I. (2009). Disgust as a disease-avoidance mechanism. *Psychological Bulletin, 135*(2), 303–321. https://doi.org/10.1037/a0014823

Ouellet-Morin, I., Odgers, C. L., Danese, A., Bowes, L., Shakoor, S., Papadopoulos, A. S., … & Arseneault, L. (2011). Blunted cortisol responses to stress signal social and behavioral problems among maltreated/bullied 12-year-old children. *Biological Psychiatry, 70*(11), 1016–1023. https://doi.org/10.1016/j.biopsych.2011.06.017

Paris, J. J., Franco, C., Sodano, R., Frye, C. A., & Wulfert, E. (2010). Gambling pathology is associated with dampened cortisol response among men and women. *Physiology & Behavior, 99*(2), 230–233. https://doi.org/10.1016/j.physbeh.2009.04.002

Pryce, C. R., Azzinnari, D., Spinelli, S., Seifritz, E., Tegethoff, M., & Meinlschmidt, G. (2011). Helplessness: A systematic translational review of theory and evidence for its relevance to understanding and treating depression. *Pharmacology & Therapeutics, 132*(3), 242–267. https://doi.org/10.1016/j.pharmthera.2011.06.006

Rizzolatti, G., & Caruana, F. (2017). How do we feel the emotions of others. *Frontiers for Young Minds, 5*(36), 10–3389. https://doi.org/10.3389/frym.2017.00036

Schroeder, K., Schuler, B. R., Kobulsky, J. M., & Sarwer, D. B. (2021). The association between adverse childhood experiences and childhood obesity: A systematic review. *Obesity Reviews*, *22*(7), e13204. https://doi.org/10.1111/obr.13204

Schwarzer, R., & Fuchs, R. (1995). Changing risk behaviors and adopting health behaviors: The role of self-efficacy beliefs. In A. Bandura (Ed.), *Self-efficacy in changing societies* (pp. 259–288). Cambridge University Press.

Schwarzer, R., & Luszczynska, A. (2006). Self-efficacy, adolescents' risk-taking behaviors, and health. In F. Pajares & T. Urdan (Eds.), *Self-efficacy beliefs of adolescents* (Vol. 5, pp. 139–159). Information Age Publishing.

Seligman, M. E., & Maier, S. F. (1967). Failure to escape traumatic shock. *Journal of Experimental Psychology, 74*(1), 1–9. https://doi.org/10.1037/h0024514

Tomoyasu, N., Bovbjerg, D. H., & Jacobsen, P. B. (1996). Conditioned reactions to cancer chemotherapy: Percent reinforcement predicts anticipatory nausea. *Physiology & Behavior*, *59*(2), 273–276. https://doi.org/10.1016/0031-9384(95)02072-1

Wicker, B., Keysers, C., Plailly, J., Royet, J. P., Gallese, V., & Rizzolatti, G. (2003). Both of us disgusted in my insula: The common neural basis of seeing and feeling disgust. *Neuron, 40*(3), 655–664.

Yu, J., Patel, R. A., Haynie, D. L., Vidal-Ribas, P., Govender, T., Sundaram, R., & Gilman, S. E. (2022). Adverse childhood experiences and premature mortality through mid-adulthood: A five-decade prospective study. *The Lancet Regional Health–Americas, 15*. https://doi.org/10.1016/j.lana.2022.100349

8 Take a Ride with Captain Trips

Psychoneuroimmunology

Infection is the most dangerous thing there is, Tom.

– Nick Andros (King, 2012, p.1126)

In my opinion, a book utilizing the works of Stephen King to explain health psychology would not be legitimate without including his epic novel *The Stand.* For one, when you ask people what their favorite Stephen King book is, most of them will invariably pick it, and it is often suggested to newbies as a good starting point for becoming a "Constant Reader." And for those of you familiar with the premise, you know that infectious disease is at the center, at least in the first part of this book. You can't talk about modern day health psychology without talking about infectious disease – so *The Stand* was made for this book (or this book was made for *The Stand*)!

Box 8.1 ***The Stand*** ⚠ **[Spoiler Alert]**

The Stand is a novel that is divided into three sections – part I is "Captain Trips," and it tells the story of how a deadly virus escaped a military research facility, eventually wiping out 99% of the world's population. Part II is "On the Border," and it tells of how the remaining 1% attempt to regroup and repair the world that is left behind. Part III, "The Stand", describes a showdown between two main groups that form in the flu's aftermath. The Free Zone and Las Vegas communities confront each other and the forces of good and evil that have arisen in the wake of Captain Trips.

For the sake of this book, we are mostly interested in Part I. As we go through *The Stand*, scientific explanations for phenomena become weaker and weaker. While *The Stand* is Stephen King's longest novel, clocking in at a whopping 472,376 words, I will attempt to provide a very brief summary of each part here.

DOI: 10.4324/9781003495994-8

Part I – Captain Trips

We begin with Charles Campion, the security guard who is able to escape the lockdown at the military research facility. Unfortunately for the world, he was exposed to Captain Trips (the manufactured super flu) before he left. While learning about Campion and his cross-country flight, we also learn about some of the main characters of the story, including Stu Redman, Frannie Goldsmith, Larry Underwood, and Nick Andros. All of them experience the collapse of the world around them in very different ways, but the one thing they have in common is that none of them succumb to the super flu. They do lose everyone they know (with a few exceptions, Frannie still has the boy she used to babysit, Harold Lauder) and must start the long and scary road to finding other survivors.

Part II

Here is where we leave behind all the mechanics of a devastating epidemic and start to consider the aftermath. Once Captain Trips has finished its destructive journey around the world, those left behind start to have vivid, recurring dreams. For some people, those dreams revolve around Mother Abigail, an extremely old woman from the Midwest who encourages people to meet her in Boulder, Colorado. For others, their dreams are inhabited by The Walkin' Dude, aka Randall Flagg, who instructs them to join him in Las Vegas, Nevada. Part II mostly consists of the journey to get to the designated locations set forth by the dreams, and adjusting to the new societies that are being built at each.

Part III

In the last part of the novel, it becomes clear that those inhabiting the Boulder Free Zone are "the good" and that those in Las Vegas are "the bad" (Who is "the ugly" you might ask? I believe that to be The Trashcan Man, who plays a pivotal role in deciding who wins the final stand-off). Recognizing that they cannot sit in Boulder ignoring the counter society being set up in Vegas, a small group of Free Zone residents set out to have a final showdown with Flagg upon instructions from Mother Abigail. Indeed, a biblical-level showdown occurs, where one faction is completely decimated. Now you only have to read about a thousand plus pages to figure out which one it is.

Welcome to the Trips

The Stand was originally published in 1978, and in 1990, it was re-released with 400 pages added that were originally cut from the first publication. For our purposes here, I will be using the "Complete and Uncut" 1990 edition. In particular, we will be focusing on the first part (Book I: Captain Trips). *The Stand* revolves around the outbreak of a very infectious, and very deadly flu, referred to throughout the book by many names: Captain Trips, A-prime, Blue Virus, and so forth. The name Blue Virus stems from the fact that it was developed at a weapons laboratory under the auspices of "Project Blue" – a secret US government war project. Despite what seems like tight security, virus 848-AB escapes the lab in the body of a military security officer named Charles Campion. This gives Charles the infamous distinction of being "Patient Zero" of this particular flu epidemic. Charles becomes the documented index case when he travels from San Diego to Texas with his wife and child, eventually crashing into Hapscomb's Texaco Station. Here, he spreads it to the unlucky gentlemen having some beer and gab during a warm June night at Hapscomb's.

Captain Trips is an extremely swift virus, and it eventually wipes out over 99% of the population – of the US for sure, but it is assumed that the entirety of the world has been affected.

Superspreaders

> There was a load of sparks.
>
> – William "Hap" Hapscomb (King, 2012, p.24)

Within the first several pages of *The Stand*, Captain Trips "superspreaders" are described. What exactly is a superspreader? In epidemiology, the term was originally coined to describe food-based outbreaks of gastrointestinal diseases (Teicher, 2023), but since the mid-20th century, it has mostly referred to air-borne respiratory illnesses. A superspreader can mean a person who is more biologically or physiologically able to transmit illness, or a person who, due to their roles in society and behavior, is more likely to spread an illness. Superspreaders can also refer to an epidemiological interpretation of the Pareto 80/20 rule,[1] which says that 20% of the population is responsible for 80% of infections (the 20% being the superspreaders). Another definition of a superspreader is someone who is the "spark" of an infectious disease outbreak (Teicher, 2023). Indeed, Hap had it right; there were a lot of sparks.

The Stand describes two types of superspreaders. The "spark" superspreader, who is of course Charles Campion. Then we have the second type of superspreader, the one that, due to their position in society and daily behavior, leads to even greater transmission of Captain Trips. Hap, who owns the Texaco station, has a cousin named Joe Bob Brentwood, with the Texas State Patrol. He stops by to visit Hap the day after Campion's crash to let them know that the health department will be stopping by to investigate. While Joe Bob gives them the heads up about the impending pathologists visit, Hap sneezes multiple times. Joe Bob suggests they close the station to make sure they are not sick. But they are, and Joe Bob leaves newly infected with Captain Trips.

Joe Bob, state patrol, then goes off to patrol the state, or his part of it at least. This is where he becomes the second type of superspreader and then infects another. Joe Bob is pulling over speeders on Highway 40 on June 18th, a few hours after fueling up at his cousins'. While we don't know how many people he came into contact during his patrol, we do know he pulled over Harry Trent, a traveling insurance salesman, another "high contract" position. Joe Bob gives Captain Trips to Trent, who over the next 48 hours gives it to over 40 people. He gave it to a majority of employees at Babe's Kwik-Eat and then gave it to a family in the parking lot who asked him for directions. Due to job responsibilities and social interactions, these were the superspreaders. If the over 40 people Trent gave it to then gave it to two to three people, well then, yes, that is how we got to 99% of the population being pretty much wiped out by July 4th.

That leaves almost 1% of the world's population alive, including Stu Redman, who was enjoying the beer and friendship at Habscombs prior to the arrival of Charles Campion. Who survived Captain Trips, and who didn't? What made some people susceptible and others not? For this, we need to look at the immune system, how it functions, and how it malfunctions, and what psychology has to do with it all.

M-O-O-N That Spells Psychoneuroimmunology: A Brief Primer

This introduces us to a subfield of health psychology called psychoneuroimmunology (PNI). PNI looks at how psychological factors, along with the nervous and immune systems, impact our health and behavior. Since the late 1970s, extensive research has shown that there are multiple pathways by which the brain, nervous system, and immune system communicate with one another. Could the findings from the field of PNI hold clues to who survived Captain Trips and who didn't?

One of the most beloved characters in *The Stand* is Tom Cullen, a kind, fun-loving, and heroic man in his 40s who survives Captain Trips. Tom has some kind of neurodevelopmental disorder, which has caused developmental delays, including an inability to read and write. When a word is a bit overwhelming for him, he often tries to spell it, but he spells everything M-O-O-N. You may hear him say something like "M - O - O - N – that spells DeeDee Packalotte." In my mind, I can hear him say "M - O - O - N – that spells Psychoneuroimmunology!" You can substitute the words if you would like to as well.

Before we move on to the specifics of PNI, it might be helpful to have a brief primer on how our immune system functions on a very basic level.

Our immune system basically consists of three lines of defense, which are needed to fight the myriad of creepy-crawlies out there (viruses, bacteria, parasites, you name it!) The more technical term for creepy-crawlies is pathogens, and they are constantly trying to invade our bodies for their own survival purposes. To fight against the pathogens, our three defenses are (1) the physical barriers that make up our body, such as our skin and mucous membranes, (2) our innate immune system, which we are born with, and (3) our adaptive immune system, which is the part of the immune system that develops and learns as we go about our lives. Captain Trips would be one of these pathogens, and we would hope that all three systems are doing their part to defend us from its ravages.

Innate Immunity (Non-Specific Immunity)

The first line of defense is pretty self-explanatory, so let's start with the innate immune system. Once something gets past our skin, whether by breaking it as a splinter might do, or finding its way through our nasal secretions into the nasal passages, our innate immune system will start a generic, non-specific campaign to fight it off. This ability is with us from the day we are born, and it is a pretty universal ability across all animals.

Key to the innate immune system are white blood cells. An important type of white blood cells are known as macrophages, and they are going to do a lot of the heavy lifting of your innate immune system. Macrophages are going to sense pathogens, approach them, and gobble them up (phage is Greek for "to eat"). When a macrophage is in the process of destroying a pathogen, it will produce a protein product called a cytokine, which sends messages back and forth between the immune system and other cells. Cytokines are inflammatory in nature – they are the reason that our wounds grow red and itchy, why we develop fevers, and a whole host of other symptoms when we are fighting off infections. Remember these cytokines – they will turn out to be very important for how the brain and immune system communicate.

Innate Immunity Is Fast

Once a foreign invader has gotten past the first line of defense, the innate immune system acts swiftly. Let's take something that happens to Nick Andros, one of the main characters in *The Stand*, as an example of how this (should) work. After a whole series of events that we can't get into here, Nick Andros, who is deaf and mute, finds himself in the role of deputy in Shoyo, Arkansas. While sitting in the station, he is ambushed by a man named Ray Booth, who had previously tried to beat Nick to death. Nick has a gun, but he is taken by such surprise that he ends up firing the gun, with the bullet grazing his leg.

While the bullet did not enter Nick's leg, it did breach the walls of his skin – causing physical damage to the tissues and creating an opening by which pathogens can enter. Once the skin has been damaged, the damaged cells will start sending chemical messages to different parts of the body to begin an innate immune response. The blood vessels near the injury will widen to increase blood flow and will become more permeable, so that immune cells can enter the tissues. These immune cells include the first responders, neutrophils, which will release substances to kill any invaders, and macrophages, which are, in essence, the clean-up crew. These cells also have the ability to release chemical signals that recruit more help. All of this can start within a few minutes, and last for hours or days, depending on the severity.

Nick does notice that this immune system response is happening – the sight of the injury turns red and hot, a result of the increased blood flow to the area. Swelling occurs as all of those immune cells leak out of the blood vessels and congregate. Then of course you have the pain that comes from all this swelling, as well as any nerve tissues that are being irritated in the process.

The hope is that our innate immune systems are working at their peak performance, and that it can easily take care of this type of injury (along with our help in restoring the barrier, via bandage). Unfortunately for Nick, it doesn't quite work out this way. First, because of a rush of adrenaline from the attack, he doesn't even know he has been injured until much later, so the wound remains open to pathogens for a significant amount of time before he bandages it up. Second, Nick has just been through a traumatizing ordeal – between getting beaten almost to death and having the super flu killing almost everyone in town – his body has been under a huge amount of stress. This stress has probably weakened his immune system (we will talk about this later in this chapter). That is why Nick's wound eventually gets infected to the point of almost killing him. His immune system could not keep the pathogens in check, so he needed to enlist the aid of an antibiotic – a medication that kills and/or inhibits the growth of bacteria in the body.

Now that you know a little bit (trust me, this is just a little bit, the immune system is VERY complicated) about the innate immune system, let's move on to acquired or adaptive immunity.

Adaptive Immunity (Specific Immunity)

Throughout *The Stand* – as the terrifying ferocity of Captain Trips becomes clear – the government tries to pacify the scared citizens by dangling the idea of an impending vaccine in front of them – this is repeated by those in power, including a very sniffly President of the United States.

Vaccines are one of the ways in which we take advantage of the amazing learning abilities of our adaptive immune system. One important thing to add here is that the pathogens we discussed above carry molecules called antigens. What happens is that when our bodies get exposed to antigens via any number of means, whether it is artificially through a vaccine, or being in your pre-school classroom with a bunch of sick classmates, it develops a memory for that antigen, so it can fight it off quickly and seamlessly the next time you are exposed to it. Thus, when you get your flu shot,[2] the idea is that when you are exposed to the flu later, you will not get sick because your adaptive immune system has learned exactly what to look for and how to fight it.

Adaptive Immunity Is Slow

While innate immunity is fast, adaptive immunity will take its time – days to weeks. This is because it is very specific, and the kind of protection it provides is long-lasting. Here is a very brief (and incomplete) description of how adaptive immunity works. First, we have cells called antigen-presenting cells (APCs) that will digest a pathogen and then take the antigen I talked about and "present" it to other immune cells. Those macrophages[3] that we discussed before can do this – they will eat up a pathogen into little pieces and then take their antigens and offer them up for other cells to see. The other cells it presents the antigen to are called helper T cells, and they are able to recognize the antigen and activate the function of two more cells – B cells and cytotoxic T cells. The B cells will then produce antibodies specific to the antigen and neutralize any surrounding pathogens, and the cytotoxic T cells will destroy the infected cells.

What makes this adaptive is that we also have Memory B and T cells – these cells remember when these specific antigens have been presented and what happened, so that when you get exposed to that pathogen and its antigen again, it can act much quicker and stronger.

Just to return to vaccines again – what vaccines do is introduce either a harmless form or a harmless level of antigen to your body so that memory cells can form. That way, when you do get exposed to the actual pathogen, you can fight it off quickly and without issue. Again, please know that this is an extremely simplified version of these processes, but I believe it is enough to get us to where we need to go next – PNI!

The Birth of PNI

How is psychology tied to the immune system? Originally, many believed there was no association between the two – that the immune system worked independently, doing its own thing without input from mind and brain. However, an amazing thing happened at the University of Rochester (go Yellowjackets, again!) in the 1970s (Pincock, 2012). Bob Ader and Nicolas Cohen were busy doing research on taste aversion in rats, and they had set up experiments where they would give rats a sweet-tasting liquid, but then pair it with an injection of a drug that would cause them to basically have an "upset stomach." Could they get the rats to not like the sweet stuff anymore through this training? Yes, they found that, but they also found something else. The drug that they were giving the rats was immunosuppressive – that is, it suppressed the regular immune response of the rat.

Ader and Cohen at one point stopped giving the rats the immunosuppressive drug but continued to feed them the sweet solution. Here is where things started to get weird. The rats who had initially been given the immunosuppressant and the sweet stuff, and who were now pretty consistently getting only the sweet stuff, started to die. They found that the more sweet stuff the rats consumed, the more likely they were to die. What was happening?

PNI, that's what! Ader and Cohen investigated further and found that after being paired with an immunosuppressant, the sweet stuff on its own actually caused an immune response – the immune system shut down, just from the sweet solution alone. The taste of sweetness was enough to instigate a series of nervous system signals that communicated to the immune system that suppression should occur. In other words, the rats tasted something sweet, the sweet taste sent a signal to the brain, which remembered that this particular taste was associated with immune suppression, and thus a series of signals was sent suppressing it once again. Ader and Cohen could behaviorally condition an immune response (just like the placebos we talked about in Chapter 4)!

This set off a tidal wave of researchers looking for the mechanism of this phenomenon – how exactly does the nervous system (including the brain) talk to the immune system, and vice versa. If taste could cause the brain to send a signal to turn off immune functioning, what other things might influence the brain, and hence immunity? Feelings of threat/stress? Other psychological phenomena?

Oh. My Bleeding Ulcer!

Another discovery that helped solidify this connection is from some Nobel prize-winning work on ulcers. Recall from Chapter 2 that we talked about the Holy Seven – on this list was peptic ulcer. This is a condition that has always been seen as psychosomatic in nature. In the 1950s, this idea certainly caught fire – imagine black and white images of high-power men in stressful situations, grabbing their midsections during high-stress work interactions, or downing bottles of Pepto Bismol and bearing down in their successful careers. This image was further ingrained into the public consciousness through the research of Brady et al. (1958), on how, when they experimentally manipulated the level of stress, a macaque monkey was more likely to develop gastrointestinal ulcers. This work was also reiterated in Seyle's stress research, which we discussed in Chapter 2.

For a very long time, ulcers such as these were seen as the domain of psychosomatic medicine, and the immune system had not entered the conversation. That is, until the 1980s, with the discovery of a bacterium called Helicobacter pylori lurking in the stomach of a majority of people with gastrointestinal ulcers. In a rare reversal of what usually happens in the mind–body debate of biomedicine versus biopsychosocial, the establishment had a hard time believing the researchers' claim that ulcers were caused by a bacterium. Ulcers being caused by stress was such an ingrained idea that it was hard for many to switch gears. Yet switching gears they did, and in 2005, the researchers, Marshall and Warren, were awarded the Nobel Prize in Medicine for their discovery of that particular creepy-crawly (Warren, 2014).

As is so often the case, most everyone switched over to the biomedicine explanation of ulcers, where if we just came up with a medical intervention for getting rid of the bacteria, ulcers would magically disappear. Except that is not how it worked out. It turns out, Helicobacter pylori is an extremely tough little bacterium, and it exists in almost all of us. How well medicines treat it is highly variable. In essence, it is very hard to get rid of, so if all of us have it, why are we not all getting ulcers?

Good question – and one in which the health psychologists and psychoneuroimmunologists were happy to comment on. The biopsychosocial people rightfully pointed out that just because the bacteria were discovered, didn't make the stress component go away. Those who experienced significant stress were still more likely to get ulcers and considering that most of us have the bacteria – maybe it was something about the psychological stress, combined with the bacteria, that led to ulcers.

And indeed, research indicates that this is the case. We can now confidently point to the fact that stress compromises the immune system. The more stressed you are, the less your immune system is able to do all the things we discussed at the beginning of this chapter (Dantzer & Kelly, 1989; Dhabhar, 2014; Morey et al., 2015). When you have a bacterium like Helicobacter pylori in your body, your immune system is able to keep it in check, under normal circumstances, so no ulcers. Yet when you start to experience psychological stress, a series of immune changes occur that make your system less able to keep Helicobacter pylori in check, and voila, ulcers! Most people now understand that it is not just one or the other – psychosomatic or biomedical – it is a combination of the two.

What does all this mean for a United States that is currently being wiped out by Captain Trips? As discussed, this super flu is highly transmissible, and just like Helicobacter pylori, pretty much everyone is exposed to it. Yet not everyone gets the symptoms when clearly exposed. This is how we can follow characters like Stu Redman, Frannie Goldsmith, Larry Underwood, Nick Andros, and many others as they try to navigate a post-epidemic world. Yet how would we know what puts you at risk for the flu and what protects you?

PNI Research – Case Control

Interestingly enough, Frannie Goldsmith and Harold Lauder, two survivors from Ogunquit, Maine, discuss what research of this nature would entail. While discussing whether or not they should leave Ogunquit, Harold mentions that there is a plaque and communicable disease center in Stovington, Vermont,[4] that might provide answers regarding Captain Trips. He states that the center may be looking for individuals who are immune. In response to Harold's idea, Frannie's inner monologue is as follows:

> They would get to Stovington, they would be taken in, tested, and out of all the tests would come some discrepancy, some difference between them and all the people that had gotten sick and died.
>
> (King, 2012, p.337)

What Frannie is describing here is a case-control study. A case-control study is observational in nature, and in most cases, it is retrospective. That is, the researchers are collecting data (the observations), and the data they are collecting is about exposures and circumstances that happened to the cases and controls prior to the disease outbreak. See Figure 8.1 for what this would look like.

This is the way a lot of research is done on diseases, especially rare diseases, or disease the pop-up quite quickly (think Covid). However, doing it this way has its problems. The biggest one is the bias inherent in trying to retrospectively recall something. Do you even remember what you ate for breakfast a few days ago, or a few weeks ago? There is so much of our life that we don't remember, especially when we don't think it is important at the time. Another thing that affects the accuracy of the retrospective report is how having the disease (or not having it) may cloud your memory or cause you to "reinterpret" exposures in light of what you are currently experiencing. So yes, Frannie is right – if she and Harold do make it to the Stovington plaque center, and people are there who are interested in what

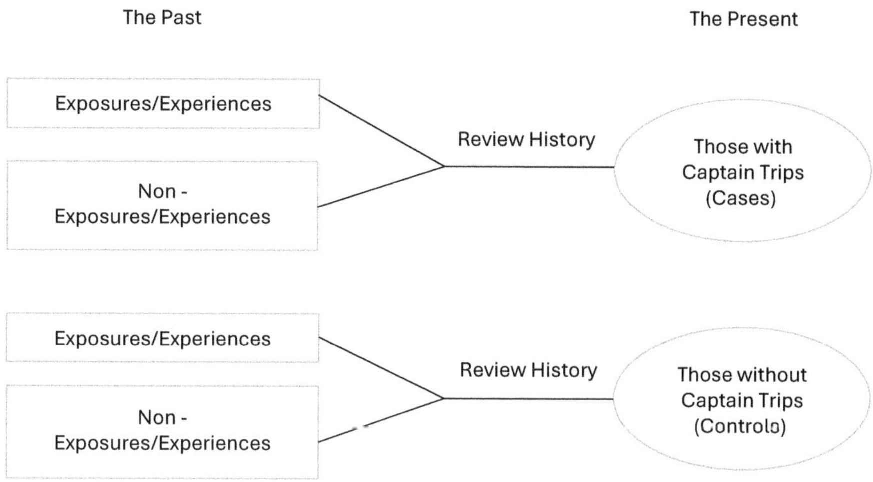

Figure 8.1 Schematic of Case-Control Study for Captain Trips.

makes one more apt to get or not get Captain Trips, they will do a retrospective case control study. Unfortunately, though, it seems as if no one has survived having Captain Trips – so getting the cases may be difficult!

There is another way you can collect data on this that controls for this retrospective bias – and that is to collect data as things are occurring, and to control when someone is exposed to an illness. This is the perfect time to introduce you to the Pittsburgh Cold Studies – a decades-long research project that looked at the biological, psychological, and social factors that make us more susceptible to infectious disease when we have been exposed.

The Pittsburgh Common Cold Studies

To tell the story of the Pittsburgh Common Cold Studies, we have to start in Salisbury, England, at the Common Cold Unit, which was founded by the British Medical Research Council in 1946. It was here that a research protocol was developed by which volunteers stayed in the unit for about ten days and were exposed to cold viruses. They were allowed to be in small groups (two to three research subjects) but were isolated from others to prevent contamination by other viruses. Most of this work was looking at different kinds of cold viruses (the first coronavirus was discovered there in 1960) and potential interventions and cures. As most of us know today, their quest for a common cold cure was unsuccessful, and the unit closed down in 1989 (Tyrrell & Fielder, 2002).

Enter Sheldon Cohen, currently Emeritus Faculty at Carnegie Mellon University in Pittsburgh (and my former PhD advisor). In the 1990s, Cohen decided to use the common cold protocol developed at the Common Cold Unit and modify it for use in determining the biopsychosocial factors that might lead people to develop infectious diseases. In this scenario, research subjects are followed for several weeks prior to being exposed to the common cold virus. This involves hard-working and dedicated graduate students (like me) calling participants nightly for two weeks and assessing their daily activities, thoughts, and feelings. We ask them things like how stressed they were that day, what they ate, how much they slept the previous night, and many other psychological and social factors, even including whether they received a hug that day.

Participants then come to the Pittsburgh version of the Common Cold Unit (the top floor of the Holiday Inn) and are quarantined there for around five days. While protocol differed slightly over the decades, you can see the timeline for the final Pittsburgh Cold Study (PCS3) in Figure 8.2. I'm using PCS3, as this was the last of the cold studies, and it was also the one that I worked on during my graduate years at Carnegie Mellon. From the years 2007 to 2011, 213 people participated in this round of cold studies.

Participants come and check into the hotel on the first night, and initial baseline measurements are collected. They then wake up in the morning and provide even more baseline data – including the main infectious disease outcomes, which are listed in Table 8.1.

An important thing to note here is that two things are being looked at as dependent variables when looking at these outcomes: (1) did the participant become infected with the virus (virus is present in nasal secretions) and (2) did they get sick (signs and symptoms) due to the infection. There are cases where participants have no indicators of infection after being exposed, there are those participants who have indicators of infection, but do not get sick, and then those who become infected and get sick because of it. From this research, we can tell which biopsychosocial factors make one more susceptible to getting infected, as well as getting sick after infection.

SCHEDULE FOR QUARANTINE DAY 0 (BASELINE MEASURES)									
4:00-5:45 pm Orientation Questionnaires Begin urine collection	DINNER	7:00-9:00 pm Temperature Blood pressure Nasal clearance	SLEEP	6:00-8:00 am Nasal wash Temperature Blood pressure Physical exam	BREAKFAST	10:00 am-noon Nasal clearance Questionnaires	LUNCH	1:00-4:00 pm Nasal clearance Temperature Blood pressure ENT exam URI symptoms	5:30 pm Collect tissues Collect urine Daily Diary: • Affect • Health practices INOCULATE VIRUS
SCHEDULE FOR QUARANTINE DAYS 1 TO 5									
	DINNER	7:00-9:00 pm Temperature Blood pressure Nasal clearance	SLEEP	6:00-8:00 am Nasal wash Temperature Blood pressure Physical exam	BREAKFAST	10:00 am-noon Nasal clearance	LUNCH	1:00-4:00 pm Nasal clearance Temperature Blood pressure ENT exam URI symptoms	5:30 pm Collect tissues Daily Diary: • Affect • Health practices

Figure 8.2 PCS3 Viral Challenge Trial Timeline.

Table 8.1 Assessments for Infection and Common Cold

Category	*Description of Measure*
Virology	
Blood (serum)	Virus-specific antibody in blood – For the cold study, a particular strain of the virus has been chosen that participants will be exposed to. At baseline, we check to make sure their adaptive immunity doesn't have a memory of being exposed to the virus before. If they are found to have prior exposure, they are disqualified from the study. Once the participant is exposed to the virus in the study, we check to see if infection memory is showing up in their immune system.
Nasal secretions	Saline solution is placed into the participants' nostrils, and they are asked to blow their noses into a cup. From these secretions, we can detect if they have been infected with the virus.
Objective cold signs	
Nasal congestion	If the participant is infected and is symptomatic, they should be experiencing nasal congestion. To test this, a nasal mucociliary clearance function test is performed. A tiny amount of sweet-tasting saccharin is placed in the nostril of the participant. They then sit quietly and breathe normally until they can taste the saccharine. The longer it takes for the saccharine to travel from the nose to their throat (where they can taste it), the more congested they are.
Mucus production	The actual amount of mucus that is being produced by the participants is calculated by having them use pre-weighed tissue paper to blow their noses. The used tissues are then collected and weighed, subtracting out the weight of the tissues.
Subject cold symptoms	Self-report – Participants fill out questionnaires about how they are feeling – including chest congestion, sinus pain, earache, fever, muscle ache, and so forth.

Now that you have a basic understanding of how some of the research in PNI works, let's look at some of the characters in *The Stand* and look at how their biopsychosocial factors influenced whether they succumbed to Captain Trips or not.

Case Study 1: Carla Goldsmith ⚠ [Spoiler Alert]

We will start with Carla Goldsmith, who is Frannie Goldsmith's mother. Carla is a strict and emotionally distant mother, who more often than not has butt heads with her independent and determined daughter. Much of this stems from trauma – when Frannie was four, her older brother Fred was killed by a drunk driver. Carla was never the same. She had also taken on a lot of responsibilities and had become very stressed when Frannie told her she was pregnant.

Carla very quickly became infected with Captain Trips, and her signs and symptoms were sudden and severe. She was an early case, so it wasn't clear yet that this wasn't isolated to just her. As Peter Goldsmith (Carla's husband, Frannie's father) put it:

> Both of us knew she's been inviting something like this, Fran. She's president of the Town Historical Committee, she's spending twenty hours a week in the library, she's secretary of the Women's Club and the Lovers of Literature Club, she's been running the March of Dimes here in town since before Fred died, and last winter she took on the Heart Fund, for good measure. On top of all that she's been trying to drum up interest in a Southern Maine Genealogical Society. She's run down, worn out. And that's part of the reason she blew up at you. Al Edmonston said was that she had the welcome mat out for the first evil germ that passed her way.
>
> (King, 2012, p.170)

Is it true? Was she just putting a doormat out for the creepy-crawlies? Research indicates that Dr. Edmonston was correct – Carla Goldsmith's immune system was probably shot. First, let's take the fact that Carla has lost a child. While it has been many years since Fred was killed, the fact that most people comment on her never being the same indicates she was not able to adapt to the loss. One systematic review and meta-analysis showed that this failure to adapt to the loss has some significant implications for immune biomarkers and resulting morbidity and mortality (Knowles et al., 2019). For example, they found lower neutrophil levels among bereaved parents, and lower antibody response to vaccinations, among other markers of immune dysfunction. More related to Carla, one study found significant immune impacts of bereaved participants when they had long-lasting dissatisfaction and confrontation avoidance after the death (Gerra et al., 2003).

This complicated grief Carla is experiencing is masked by her overinvolvement in community activities and her overinvolvement with her daughter. I think that her big-blow out with Frannie, which causes Frannie to move out, demonstrates how much Carla is feeling that the things around her are out of control. This is classic perceived stress – when you feel like life's demands and challenges are outweighing your resources, energies, and capabilities. The most widely used measure of perceived stress is the Perceived Stress Scale (PSS; Cohen et al., 1994). Here are the questions from the PSS-10, which was used in PSC3 Cold Study (Table 8.2):

To score the PSS-10, you would add up the points based on how each question was answered. Higher scores are indicative of more perceived

Table 8.2 Ten-Item Perceived Stress Scale

Question	*Never*	*Almost Never*	*Sometimes*	*Fairly Often*	*Very Often*
In the last month, how often have you been upset because of something that happened unexpectedly	0	1	2	3	4
In the last month, how often have you felt that you were unable to control the important things in your life?	0	1	2	3	4
In the last month, how often have you felt nervous and "stressed"?	0	1	2	3	4
In the last month, how often have you felt confident about your ability to handle your personal problems?	4	3	2	1	0
In the last month, how often have you felt that things were going your way?	4	3	2	1	0
In the last month, how often have you found that you could not cope with all the things that you had to do?	0	1	2	3	4
In the last month, how often have you been able to control irritations in your life?	4	3	2	1	0
In the last month, how often have you felt that you were on top of things?	4	3	2	1	0
In the last month, how often have you been angered because of things that happened that were outside of your control?	0	1	2	3	4
In the last month, how often have you felt difficulties were piling up so high that you could not overcome them?	0	1	2	3	4

stress. Looking at this, I think that Carla Goldsmith would have scored extremely high at the time she got sick.

This would be predicted by the cold studies. When participants had high perceived stress scores, they were more likely to get infected with the virus, and then they were also more likely to get a clinical cold (Cohen et al., 1991, 1993). They also looked at specific kinds of stressors, and they found that interpersonal problems with family or friends significantly increased the risk of getting a cold after exposure (Cohen et al., 1998). This would include her falling out with her only surviving child, Frannie, and her argument with her husband because of it.

Finally, Carla's lack of warmth and negative rigidity may have also made her more immunologically susceptible to Captain Trips. Remember how people were interviewed for several weeks prior to cold exposure and quarantine? It was found that people who used more positive words (lively, pleased, at ease, etc.) to describe their mood on those days were much less likely to get the cold than people with low rates of using those words (Cohen et al., 2003b). I actually can't imagine Carla using any of those words in daily life, so it is no surprise if this placed her at risk as well.

The result of all of this is that we had to say goodbye to Carla early in the novel. Unfortunately, her husband Peter dies as well (again, this could be the immune system effects of bereavement), and Frannie is left alone, at least until Harold Lauder comes around to see his favorite babysitter.

Case Study 2: Stu Redman

Now we will turn to some protective factors as Stu has made it through the epidemic – despite almost being left behind in quarantine to die (or be killed!). What characteristics of Stu help his immune system protect him so well?

The first thing I will say about Stu is that I think he is a pretty sociable guy. Here he is chatting away with his friends at Hap's Texaco station. Then he meets Glen Batemen, chatting up him and Kojak (see Box 8.3). Then it is Harold and Frannie, and then all of a sudden, he is the de facto leader of The Free Zone. This sociability – the ability to seek others out and be agreeable in interactions – was found to be a protective factor in the common cold studies (Cohen et al., 2003a). The sociability of a person was assessed using three measures: levels of extraversion, levels of agreeableness, and a positive relationship style. Those who scored high in this measure were much less likely to get the cold after exposure. Score one for Stu!

Another characteristic of Stu would be his resilience and self-efficacy (similar to what we discussed in terms of Gordie in Chapter 7). Stu has had his wife die of cancer, he watched all his friends die of Captain Trips, and then he had to fight his way out of quarantine when it was clear he was the only one who had survived the Trips. Yet he was still roaming the New England countryside looking for companions, keeping his chin up. He is able to overcome adversity, and he is also able to recognize what needs to get done, and then he does it.

This bodes well for his immune system. In a fairly recent review paper, it was found that resilience impacts the immune system through several pathways, including reducing the impact of stress, increasing personal control, and improving social support (Dantzer et al., 2018). For self-efficacy, one experimental study demonstrated that the more self-efficacy one reported, the better the immune outcomes when faced with an experimental stressor (Wiedenfeld et al., 1990).

All of these factors indicate to me that Stu Redman has a well-functioning immune system. Thanks to that, and a little help from Kojak and Tom Cullen, he is able to survive his desert ordeal – but I won't give away any more than that!

Box 8.2 Stu Redman and Whitecoat Hypertension

When it is discovered that Stu Redman is just not getting Captain Trips, he falls under the scrutiny of the doctors and researchers at the Stovington Plague and Infectious Disease Center. Frustrated by the lack of information he receives as he is kept quarantined in a small room, he decides to refuse to cooperate until they tell him what is going on. When a nurse enters his room to take a blood pressure reading, he refuses, and the issue is not pressed upon. Stu reflects on this and realizes that a blood pressure reading taken under duress would not be accurate. What he is describing here is a perfect real-world example of health psychology in action. This idea that you would not get an accurate blood pressure reading in a doctor's office, or other clinical settings, is often referred to as "whitecoat hypertension." When someone is at the doctor's and their blood pressure reading is high, about 15–30% of those high readings are simply due to being in an office. A major factor in experiencing whitecoat hypertension is anxiety – the more anxious the patient is over the health care interaction, the higher their blood pressure (Franklin et al., 2013). One way to eliminate these whitecoat effects is to improve communication, trust, and empathy between doctor and patient (Cobos et al., 2015). Unfortunately for Stu, I don't think his doctors are interested in improving their bedside manner!

Case Study 3: Sheriff John Baker ⚠ [Spoiler Alert]

I love the character of John Baker, and how he and his wife take care of Nick Andros when he is at his lowest. As such, it hurts my heart a bit to have him here as one of the high-risk cases. He is a highly sociable and good-natured person – but he has a few issues that put him at risk for infectious disease – his career and his sleep habits.

We have already talked in detail about the health of law enforcement officers (LEOs), especially when it comes to mental health, cardiovascular disease, and cancer. One of the big factors of LEOs' work is that they work in shifts, and John Baker pulls a lot of overnight shifts. Researchers found that this shift work among police officers led to overzealous immune reactions – increased levels of white blood cells, including neutrophils (Wirth et al., 2017). This dysregulation of the immune system – where your body is mounting an immune response for no acute reason – is highly associated with a whole host of diseases. One study that looked at self-reports of head and chest colds found that shift workers were 20% more likely to report having a cold when compared to those who worked during the day (Prather & Carroll, 2021). This shift work aspect of John Baker's profession brings us to an even bigger risk factor – sleep.

We will go over sleep in-depth in the next chapter, but we will briefly review the cold study findings here. The study that was just mentioned by Prather and Carroll also found that when compared to people who get the recommended seven to eight hours of sleep, those sleeping five or fewer hours were 44% more likely to report head or chest colds. John Baker fits in this sleep less than five hours category – he states that he can't get any more than three or four hours a night. Using data from the cold studies, a gradient effect was found for sleep efficiency (the amount of time you spend in bed actually sleeping) – where those getting the lowest amounts of sleep efficiency have the highest percentage of colds, and those with the most efficiency the lowest percentage (Cohen et al., 2009). They also found that those with less than seven hours of sleep were 2.94 times more likely to get a cold than those with eight or more.

In these studies, self-report was used, and sometimes people can be inaccurate about their own sleep schedules and efficiencies. Thus, the question was asked again with the addition of actigraphy data, which was gathered by a watch-type device worn on the wrist that measures movement (Prather et al., 2015). Forty-five percent of those who slept less than five hours got the cold, whereas only about 17% of those with seven or more hours did. Again, as the amount of sleep decreases, the chances of getting a cold increase.

Poor Sheriff John Baker, his immune system had really taken a beating from his lack of sleep, and there was no way he was going to survive Captain Trips. Luckily, he left Nick Andros better than when he found him, so we can be thankful for that.

Case Study 4: Glendon Pequod "Glen" Bateman

While Glen is a 57-year-old widower, which puts him at certain disadvantages, he has a few protective factors I would like to very briefly discuss. The biggest one is his education – Glen has three degrees – one bachelor's and two master's. He is also a sociology professor who seems pretty well off. As such, I am going to place him as high socioeconomic status (SES). Maybe not as high as you can go, but definitely in an advantageous spot. In one review and meta-analysis, researchers looked at SES and the outcomes from two different influenza pandemics: 1918 and 2009 (Mamelund et al., 2021). In analyzing all of the studies, they found that low SES was associated with an average 40% higher rate of influenza. They also found that in controlled studies, low SES was associated with worse influenza outcomes.

Along with his positive disposition, sociability, and his new dog Kojak (see Box 8.3), I would say Glen is well protected from the virus.

Box 8.3 The Real Hero of *The Stand* – Kojak

For many who read *The Stand*, the real hero is Kojak – the Irish Setter that Glen Bateman stumbles upon in the early days of the Captain Trips epidemic. Despite being left behind, attacked by wolves, and left stranded with Stu Redman, he remains steadfastly loyal, providing the humans around him with hope, warmth (both physical and emotional), and rabbits.

For those of us who love dogs, this comes as no surprise. Kojak helps the survivors continue to survive, and the benefits of pets, especially dogs, are well-known in health psychology. For example, multiple studies have shown that pets can reduce stress and consequently lower blood pressure. In one study (Friedmann et al., 2011), pet ownership was shown to help people with long-term recovery from myocardial infarctions (heart attacks). What they found was that pet owners were 67% less likely to die than non-pet owners. This study also indicated that the key benefit of having a pet was the reduction in depression, which often occurs after someone has suffered a heart attack (Desai et al., 2025; Thombs, 2006).

While pet ownership in general can reduce depression and its physical consequences, dog ownership in particular works directly on physical health through increased exercise that occurs when walking dogs (Cutt et al., 2007).

But perhaps one of the greatest benefits of dogs is the way in which they non-judgmentally support us. Even after Glen left Kojak behind, the dog provides unconditional love for him, Stu, and the others. One of my favorite studies (Allen et al., 1991) demonstrated that when it comes to the stress of being evaluated, the presence of your dog is much more beneficial than the presence of your human best friend. The researchers looked at 45 adult women who were asked to perform a standard stress task in the lab (with just the researcher present), and then do it again at their home with the addition of their pet dog being present, their female friend, or neither.

In this case, the stressful task was what we call serial subtraction. Subjects are given a four-digit number, let's say it is 1325, and are asked to count backward by 7s (1318, 1311, 1304, 1297, etc.). While the women were doing these stressful tasks, their pulse rate, skin conductance, and blood pressure were taken. When doing the stressful task in the lab, all women showed increased heart rate, skin conductance, and blood pressure, meaning they had a physiological stress response. However, in the home condition, the women who performed the tasks with their pet dog present did not show a significant stress response. Women who were with only the experimenter showed a significant stress response, and those who were with their female friend showed the greatest increases in heart rate, skin conductance, and blood pressure.

In essence, having your dog there meant no stress response to the task, whereas having your female friend there meant an even larger stress response than normal. The researchers concluded that the dog was a non-judgmental other offering support and making the task less stressful, whereas the human companion came with the potential for judgment, making the person even more stressed out. When Stu Redman said to, Kojak, "Say, that's a good dog" (King, 2012, p.757) – he had the science to back it up!

We have to leave this chapter here, even though there is so much more to say about the immune system and *The Stand.* The amount I left out about both absolutely dwarfs what I have said here. But we will save that for another day, and another book.

The Stand

Novel: King, S. (1990). *The Stand: The Complete & Uncut Edition.* Doubleday.

Audiobook: King, S. (1990). *The Stand: The Complete & Uncut Edition* (Narrated by Grover Gardner) [Audiobook]. Recorded Books. https://www.recordedbooks.com/title-details/9781980069746

TV Miniseries*:*

Garris, M. (Director). (1994). *The Stand* [TV miniseries]. Laurel Entertainment; ABC.

Cavell, B. (Executive Producer). (2020). *The Stand* [TV miniseries]. CBS Studios; Mosaic Media Group; Vertigo Entertainment.

Further Explorations

1 There are many other case studies that can be done with characters from *The Stand*. Do your own case study using either the book or one of the miniseries. Make sure you fill out the PSS-10 for each case you look at. What connections can you make between the character and their immunity?

2 In 2011, the researchers responsible for the Pittsburgh Cold Studies developed the Common Cold Project (https://www.cmu.edu/common-cold-project/). This is a repository of all 25 years' worth of cold study data. On the website, you can look at all the different cold study trials and see a detailed list of all variables collected during each wave of the study. Can you come up with some good questions regarding biopsychosocial influences on common cold susceptibility? Granted, many questions have already been asked and answered from these data – but with so much data collected, there is still much more we can ask! And all of the data is available to the public, so once you come up with your questions/hypothesis, the potential for testing them is in your hands. This could make for a great class research project, or senior honors thesis. Details on how to get the data are available on the website.

3 One of the most moving chapters of *The Stand* has nothing to do with any of the main characters. Book 1, Chapter 38, discusses the deaths that occur due to a "second epidemic" – that is, one in which the number of deaths by reasons other than infectious disease skyrockets. Much of what happens to people in this chapter is reflected in the leading causes of death in the United States (https://www.cdc.gov/nchs/fastats/leading-causes-of-death.htm). How does health psychology attempt to prevent some of the deaths that happen in the "second epidemic"? Pick one of the unfortunate characters in this chapter and investigate the primary, secondary, or tertiary prevention strategies that health psychologists employ to ensure what happens to them doesn't happen to others. How do you think the stress of the "first epidemic" influenced the outcomes for the people in the second epidemic?

Notes

1 The Pareto rule is named after the 19th century Italian economist Vilfredo Pareto, who observed that in Italy, 80% of the wealth was owned by 20% of the population (Persky, 1992).

2 Flu shots are tricky ones, because there are so many different flu variants out there. Every year scientists will collect and analyze flu virus samples from around the world, and they determine which ones are circulating the quickest and causing the most illness. They then make recommendation for which strains should be selected for the vaccine. For this season (I am getting my shot in a few weeks), the FDA recommended to vaccine manufacturers that the flu vaccine should include HIN1, H3N2, and B/Victoria lineage (FDA, https://www.fda.gov/vaccines-blood-biologics/influenza-vaccine-composition-2025-2026-us-influenza-season). Thus, when you get a flu shot, it does not protect you from all the flu variants, only those deemed as posing the most potential risk.

3 Macrophages are my favorite part of the immune system. They are amazing.

4 This is the same Stovington where Jack Torrence taught English in *The Shining*.

Bibliography

Allen, K. M., Blascovich, J., Tomaka, J., & Kelsey, R. M. (1991). Presence of human friends and pet dogs as moderators of autonomic responses to stress in women. *Journal of Personality and Social Psychology, 61*(4), 582. https://doi.org/10.1037/0022-3514.61.4.582

Brady, J. V. (1958). Ulcers in "executive" monkeys. *Scientific American, 199*(4), 95–103. https://doi.org/10.1038/scientificamerican1058-95

Cobos, B., Haskard-Zolnierek, K., & Howard, K. (2015). White coat hypertension: Improving the patient–health care practitioner relationship. *Psychology Research and Behavior Management, 8*, 133–141. https://doi.org/10.2147/PRBM.S61192

Cohen, S., Doyle, W. J., Alper, C. M., Janicki-Deverts, D., & Turner, R. B. (2009). Sleep habits and susceptibility to the common cold. *Archives of Internal Medicine, 169*(1), 62–67. https://doi.org/10.1001/archinternmed.2008.505

Cohen, S., Doyle, W. J., Turner, R., Alper, C. M., & Skoner, D. P. (2003a). Sociability and susceptibility to the common cold. *Psychological Science, 14*(5), 389–395.

Cohen, S., Doyle, W. J., Turner, R. B., Alper, C. M., & Skoner, D. P. (2003b). Emotional style and susceptibility to the common cold. *Psychosomatic Medicine, 65*(4), 652–657. https://doi.org/10.1097/01.PSY.0000077508.57784.DA

Cohen, S., Frank, E., Doyle, W. J., Skoner, D. P., Rabin, B. S., & Gwaltney Jr, J. M. (1998). Types of stressors that increase susceptibility to the common cold in healthy adults. *Health Psychology, 17*(3), 214–223.

Cohen, S., Kamarck, T., & Mermelstein, R. (1994). Perceived stress scale. *Measuring Stress: A Guide for Health and Social Scientists, 10*(2), 1–2.

Cohen, S., Tyrrell, D. A., & Smith, A. P. (1991). Psychological stress and susceptibility to the common cold. *New England Journal of Medicine, 325*(9), 606–612.

Cohen, S., Tyrrell, D. A., & Smith, A. P. (1993). Negative life events, perceived stress, negative affect, and susceptibility to the common cold. *Journal of Personality and Social Psychology, 64*(1), 131–140.

Cutt, H., Giles-Corti, B., Knuiman, M., & Burke, V. (2007). Dog ownership, health and physical activity: A critical review of the literature. *Health & Place, 13*(1), 261–272. https://doi.org/10.1016/j.healthplace.2006.01.003

Dantzer, R., Cohen, S., Russo, S. J., & Dinan, T. G. (2018). Resilience and immunity. *Brain, Behavior, and Immunity, 74*, 28–42. https://doi.org/10.1016/j.bbi.2018.08.010

Dantzer, R., & Kelley, K. W. (1989). Stress and immunity: An integrated view of relationships between the brain and the immune system. *Life Sciences, 44*(26), 1995–2008.

Desai, H. N., Wali, P., Desai, K., Bilgaiyan, R., & Raval, R. (2025). The heart-mind connection: A systematic review xxploring the bidirectional relationship between myocardial infarction and depression. *American Journal of Psychology and Brain Studies, 2*(3), 108–116.

Dhabhar, F. S. (2014). Effects of stress on immune function: The good, the bad, and the beautiful. *Immunologic Research, 58*(2), 193–210. https://doi.org/10.1007/s12026-014-8517-0

Franklin, S. S., Thijs, L., Hansen, T. W., O'brien, E., & Staessen, J. A. (2013). White-coat hypertension: New insights from recent studies. *Hypertension, 62*(6), 982–987. https://doi.org/10.1161/HYPERTENSIONAHA.113.01275

Friedmann, E., Thomas, S. A., & Son, H. (2011). Pets, depression and long-term survival in community living patients following myocardial infarction. *Anthrozoös, 24*(3), 273–285. https://doi.org/10.2752/175303711X13045914865268

Gerra, G., Monti, D., Panerai, A. E., Sacerdote, P., Anderlini, R., Avanzini, P., … & Franceschi, C. (2003). Long-term immune-endocrine effects of bereavement: Relationships with anxiety levels and mood. *Psychiatry Research, 121*(2), 145–158. https://doi.org/10.1016/S0165-1781(03)00255-5

King, S. (2012). *The Stand.* Random House. https://www.amazon.com/dp/B0078XGJXO

Knowles, L. M., Ruiz, J. M., & O'Connor, M. F. (2019). A systematic review of the association between bereavement and biomarkers of immune function. *Psychosomatic Medicine, 81*(5), 415–433. https://doi.org/10.1097/PSY.0000000000000693

Mamelund, S. E., Shelley-Egan, C., & Rogeberg, O. (2021). The association between socioeconomic status and pandemic influenza: Systematic review and meta-analysis. *PLOS One, 16*(9), e0244346. https://doi.org/10.1371/journal.pone.0244346

Morey, J. N., Boggero, I. A., Scott, A. B., & Segerstrom, S. C. (2015). Current directions in stress and human immune function. *Current Opinion in Psychology, 5*, 13–17. https://doi.org/10.1016/j.copsyc.2015.03.007

Overmier, J. B., & Murison, R. (2013). Restoring psychology's role in peptic ulcer. *Applied Psychology: Health and Well-Being, 5*(1), 5–27. https://doi.org/10.1111/j.1758-0854.2012.01076.x

Persky, J. (1992). Retrospectives: Pareto's law. *Journal of Economic Perspectives, 6*(2), 181–192.

Pincock, S. (2012). Robert Ader. *The Lancet, 379*(9813), 308.

Prather, A. A., & Carroll, J. E. (2021). Associations between sleep duration, shift work, and infectious illness in the United States: Data from the National Health Interview Survey. *Sleep Health, 7*(5), 638–643. https://doi.org/10.1016/j.sleh.2021.05.004

Prather, A. A., Janicki-Deverts, D., Hall, M. H., & Cohen, S. (2015). Behaviorally assessed sleep and susceptibility to the common cold. *Sleep, 38*(9), 1353–1359. https://doi.org/10.5665/sleep.4968

Teicher, A. (2023). Super-spreaders: A historical review. *The Lancet Infectious Diseases, 23*(10), e409–e417. https://doi.org/10.1016/S1473-3099(23)00183-4

Thombs, B. D., Bass, E. B., Ford, D. E., Stewart, K. J., Tsilidis, K. K., Patel, U., … & Ziegelstein, R. C. (2006). Prevalence of depression in survivors of acute myocardial infarction: Review of the evidence. *Journal of General Internal Medicine, 21*(1), 30–38. https://doi.org/10.1111/j.1525-1497.2005.00269.x

Tyrrell, D. A. J., & Fielder, M. (2002). *Cold wars: The fight against the common cold.* Oxford University Press.

Warren, J. R. (2014). *Helicobacter–The ease and difficulty of a new discovery.* World Scientific.

Wiedenfeld, S. A., O'Leary, A., Bandura, A., Brown, S., Levine, S., & Raska, K. (1990). Impact of perceived self-efficacy in coping with stressors on components of the immune system. *Journal of Personality and Social Psychology, 59*(5), 1082. https://doi.org/10.1037/0022-3514.59.5.1082

Wirth, M. D., Andrew, M. E., Burchfiel, C. M., Burch, J. B., Fekedulegn, D., Hartley, T. A., … & Violanti, J. M. (2017). Association of shiftwork and immune cells among police officers from the buffalo cardio-metabolic occupational police stress study. *Chronobiology International, 34*(6), 721–731. https://doi.org/10.1080/07420528.2017.1316732

9 The Nightmare of *Insomnia*

The Importance of Sleep

"The Incredible Insomniac of Harris Avenue"

While there are so many great Stephen King characters, my personal favorite is Ralph Roberts, the protagonist of the 1994 novel *Insomnia.* Referring to himself as "The Incredible Insomniac of Harris Avenue" (King, 2016, p.60), Ralph struggles with sleep, grief, growing old, and, of course, something of the supernatural variety (see Box 9.1 for summary). In this chapter, we will focus on the health psychology of sleep and take a few detours to discuss the grief and social connectedness that Ralph experiences in addition to his insomnia. I love Ralph Roberts, and I love sleep – and I hope by the end of this chapter you will too!

Box 9.1 *Insomnia*

Like many of Stephen King's books and short stories, *Insomnia* is a novel set in Derry, Maine. Published in 1994, it tells the story of Ralph Roberts, a 70-year-old man who has recently lost his wife and is experiencing an increasingly severe bout of insomnia. He is also dealing with the actions of his paranoid neighbor, Ed Deepneau, including Ed's recent severe beating of his wife, Helen, in front of their toddler, Natalie. Thankfully, Helen leaves Ed – but that does not stop his ever-increasing delusions around a man named The Crimson King, and the King's demand that he fights off "Centurians," of which Ralph has been labeled.

Ralph is also surrounded by his two closest friends, Bill McGovern and Lois Chasse, as well as a group of elderly Derry residents, known as the "Harris Avenue Old Crocks." The talk among all of these Derry residents is the approaching arrival of author/activist Susan Day, who will be giving a pro-choice talk at the Derry Civic Center. Susan Day has been targeted by Ed Deepneau and other right-to-lifers as public enemy number one, and Derry seems to be rife with constant turmoil around her and the women's center she is raising money for.

⚠ **[Spoiler Alert]** All this is happening against the backdrop of Ralph's increasing insomnia, and he finds out that Lois is experiencing sleep difficulties

DOI: 10.4324/9781003495994-9

as well. Along with the sleep difficulties, the two of them are also experiencing extra sensory phenomena – particularly auras around people and "balloon strings" above their heads that seem to indicate life expectancy. Ralph and Lois are also able to see Clotho and Lechesis – entities who look like small bald doctors – and that seem to show up when people in Derry pass away.

Clotho and Lechesis recruit Ralph and Lois to help them with the third of their trio – Atropos – who has gone rogue. Atropos is actually the one who is feeding Ed Deepneau the ideas and images of the Crimson King, and who has guided Ed to get rid of Susan Day and all "Centurians" who kill unborn babies. Ed is planning a devastating attack on the Derry Civic Center, and it is up to Ralph and Lois to stop him. In an amazing sequence of events, Ralph does indeed stop Ed, and saves the most important person in the Civic Center – not Susan Day, but Patrick Danville (see *The Dark Tower* series – and may you have long days and pleasant nights).

Soon after, both Ralph and Lois see a resolution to their insomnia and extrasensory perception, and they end up getting married. As the years go by, the memories of their sleepless nights and interactions with Clotho and Lechesis disappear. They live happily ever after … until they don't.

What Is Sleep?

Before we get into the sleep troubles of Ralph Roberts, it might be a good idea to discuss some of the science of sleep. The beauty of *Insomnia* is that it provides a lot of this information within the story, thanks to Joe Wyzer, the pharmacist Ralph runs into when seeking over-the-counter sleep aids at the Rite-Aid. Over coffee at the local diner, Joe imparts his knowledge of sleep to Ralph, who listens with rapt attention.

> "Sleep is the overlooked hero and the poor man's physician"– Joe Wyzer.
> (King, 2016, p.139)

Joe stresses to Ralph that sleep is fundamental for our survival, up there with water, food, and shelter. And of course, he is 100% correct (Grandner, 2016).

Circadian Rhythms

We spend about 1/3 of our lives sleeping, so we know it is important. It is part of an ingrained pattern within our biological framework called our circadian rhythms. Our bodies have all sorts of rhythms that keep us functioning for survival – these include ultradian and infradian rhythms, along with the circadian. Ultradian rhythms refer to any repeating patterns that occur in a span of time less than 24 hours. For example, the hormonal cycles of leptin and ghrelin, which tell us when we are hungry and when we are full, are ultradian in nature. Infradian, on the other hand, refers to cycles that span time period longer than 24 hours, such as menstrual cycles and hibernation in certain animals. Circadian rhythms are the ones that occur within an approximately 24-hour time span,[1] and they include all the physiological and biological processes incorporated in our sleep/wake cycle.

Circadian rhythms are reactive to zeitgebers, literally translated to "time giver." Many things we are exposed to in our everyday life can be a zeitgeber – the temperature, what we are eating, what medications we take (see the discussion below of folk remedies for insomnia – many of these are trying to be zeitgebers). Yet the most potent zeitgeber is light, and it is the one that we, and a majority of the cells in our body, are reactive to (Meyer et al., 2022).

While we all know that our eyes are sensitive to light, did you know that in our eyes, we have cells that are especially sensitive to certain kinds of light, and they have nothing to do with creating a visual image? These specialized eye cells contain melanopsin, a protein photoreceptor that is involved in sending light signals to the suprachiasmatic nucleus (SCN), located in the hypothalamus (Duda et al., 2020). The SCN is referred to as our master circadian clock, and it uses these light signals from the eye to figure out when it is night and when it is day, when we should be asleep, and when we should be awake (Patton & Hastings, 2018).

When the SCN is no longer receiving light signals, it will send a message to the pineal gland to start producing melatonin – the hormone that makes us sleepy. Later, when the SCN starts to pick up light signals signifying morning, it will produce cortisol, which will begin to rise before you wake up, but hit maximum levels about 30–45 minutes after waking (Stalder et al., 2025). This is known as the cortisol awakening response, and it is just as important as melatonin in regulating the circadian sleep – wake cycle.

Circadian rhythms are important to understand because a lot of our sleep troubles come from a misalignment of our sleep schedules with the light signals. This is especially true of shift workers, those who travel across time zones frequently, and those who expose themselves to too much light (cell phones, ahem) around their preferred bedtimes (you know who you are!).

For Ralph Roberts, his age may be playing a role in how his circadian rhythms are functioning. For example, research shows that when you compare older adults to younger adults, older adults have fewer fluctuations in melatonin, and they are not exposed to it for a long time. This may be why older people in general become morning people – they are much more likely to get up early than younger people (Hood & Amir, 2017). Older people also see decreased amounts of SCN firing, as well as cortisol, which is assumed to be a natural function of aging. Thus, Ralph Roberts was probably already experiencing the age-related changes in sleep prior to the onset of his insomnia.

Sleep Stages

Once the melatonin has kicked in, we become sleepy and get into bed, ready for our eight hours of sleep – what happens next? This is when we start to cycle through the stages of sleep. There are two types of sleep, non-rapid eye movement (NREM) sleep and rapid eye movement (REM) sleep. You will cycle through the types throughout the night, but you will start off with NREM sleep. You get most of your NREM sleep in the beginning of your eight hours, and it has been found to be key in physical restoration – repairing the cells (muscle, immune, etc.) that you have used throughout the day. NREM has three main stages – Stage 1 is light sleep, and here is where you can be easily awakened. It doesn't last too long before you head into Stage 2. At this stage, you are going to experience a lot of physiological changes – your temperature falls and your heart rate slows. From here, you will go to Stage 3 (sometimes divided into Stages 3 and 4), where you will then be in slow-wave sleep (SWS). SWS is the deepest sleep, and it will be very hard for you to wake up. This is where that physical restoration occurs, so it is hugely important for your biological functioning.

After you have gone into SWS, you will eventually cycle back through Stage 2, then Stage 1, until you start REM, which will occur about 90 minutes after you first went to sleep. It is called REM sleep because your eyes will start rapidly moving, and your brain waves will look almost like you are awake; however, most of your muscles are in a form of paralysis, so you don't move. This is the part of sleep where you will be doing more of the mental work – your brain processes emotions, consolidates memories, and solves problems. This is also the state where most people report having vivid dreams. You will do the majority of your REM sleep at the end of the night, so it is important to get a full night's sleep so you can be both restored physically and mentally.

You will cycle through these stages throughout the night, with SWS occurring longer in the early cycles, and REM being more prolific in the later cycles. Many people who are not getting enough sleep have no problem with their NREM requirements – what they are missing out on is the REM needed to be fully functioning the next day. This is where Ralph Roberts' problems come into play – he is able to get to sleep at night, and he is probably cycling through his NREM without issue. However, since he is constantly waking up early and not able to get back to sleep, he is missing out on important late-cycle REM. This is the reason he is experiencing some short-term memory loss, like his inability to remember eating the last Lipton Cup-A-Soup.

Some of Ralph's sleep problems may be just due to age. Our sleep cycles and patterns don't stay the same throughout our entire lives. When we are first born, we need a lot of sleep, and we haven't yet figured out that circadian rhythm thing. We slowly need less sleep as we grow, but we still need the most during our developmental years. In our preteens, we need to have about 9–11 hours, 8–10 when we are teenagers, and then 7–9 hours from the ages of 18–25. Seven to nine hours is also recommended for adults until the age of about 65. For people Ralph's age, the recommendation is 7–8 hours, but this is an area where there is not as much consensus (Hirshkowitz et al., 2015). Five to six hours may be appropriate for this age group, as SWS and REM sleep durations tend to decline with age (Li et al., 2022).

Still, Ralph Roberts seems to be getting much less than that. We should not just assume that his sleep problems are age-related. There may be other factors (see Box 9.2 for one possible explanation) and considerations. What we should do next is investigate a little bit more by having Ralph fill out the most widely used questionnaires about sleep – The Pittsburgh Sleep Quality Index (PSQI).[2]

Box 9.2 Ralph's Grief

When we first meet Ralph, he is living through the last months of his wife's life, as she slowly dies from brain cancer. It is about six months after her passing that he starts to experience debilitating sleep problems. Could these sleep problems stem from grief over his wife's death? One systematic review (Lancel et al., 2020) suggests that it is something to consider. When searching through 85 scientific articles that looked at over 12,000 participants, they found that there were high rates of sleep disturbances among bereaved people. Another study, which looked at actigraphy[3]-assessed sleep, as well as the PSQI, found that those who were experiencing grief had low sleep efficiency and poor self-rated sleep quality (de Feijter et al., 2021).

However, much of the research indicates that sleep problems are mostly associated with complicated grief (e.g., Milic et al., 2019). We call grief complicated when it lasts longer than what is considered normal by societal standards and when it impairs the person's daily functioning. This is not just "normal" grieving – it can be quite severe, and it involves preoccupation with the deceased, and a disbelief around the loss. The person also has a hard time accepting a future without the person (Shear, 2015). This does not sound like Ralph Roberts to me – while his grief is palpable, it is not to a point where it prevents him from performing daily activities or planning for the future.

The PSQI

The PSQI (pronounced piskey) was developed by Dan Buysse and colleagues at the University of Pittsburgh in the late 1980s. It is a self-report questionnaire that asks people about their sleep over the last month in order to get a better understanding of the quality of their sleep. The higher your score, the better your sleep. The beauty of the PSQI is that it can be used in both a research and clinical setting – to help figure out if individuals are having good or bad sleep (it cannot diagnose sleep disorders), and to figure out the known risks and outcomes associated with sleep.

In order to get at certain sleep parameters, the PSQI asks ten questions, many with sub-questions following. The first four questions are very general: in the past month, when have you usually gone to bed, how long has it taken you to fall asleep, when have you usually gotten up, and how many hours of actual sleep did you get. It then asks the frequency of certain situations and behaviors that have occurred over the last month, such as: not being able to get to sleep within the first 30 minutes of laying down, waking up in the middle of the night or early in the morning, getting up for bathroom breaks, difficulty breathing, coughing and snoring, too cold, too hot, bad dreams, pain, and other (which the person will specify). It asks the person to provide their own rating of their sleep quality, if they have taken anything medicinal to help with sleep, and if they have problems staying awake during daily activities. It also assesses whether their sleep is affecting their motivation.

Lastly, it asks about sleeping partners – since the presence of another while sleeping can greatly impact your own sleep quality, especially if they snore. The PSQI assesses whether the person's roommate or bed partner (if they have one): snores loudly, takes long pauses between breaths,[4] jerks or twitches legs while sleeping,[5] is disoriented or confused while they sleep,[6] or has other forms of restlessness. And yes, while these symptoms in the roommate or partner are concerning and should be checked out – the PSQI is interested in the sleep of the person answering, and these issues could be impacting them greatly.

Once you get the person's responses on the PSQI, you can calculate some important components of sleep:

Subjective Sleep Quality – how the person is perceiving their own sleep
Sleep Latency – the average time it takes the person to fall asleep
Sleep Duration – the total hours of sleep per night they are getting
Sleep Efficiency – this is calculated by taking the total time they spend asleep and dividing it by the total time they spend in bed. Example – if you have slept seven hours, but it took you 30 minutes to get to sleep, and you were awake for an hour during the night, then your sleep efficiency is 7 divided by 8.5 = approximately 82% sleep efficiency (not good!)
Daytime Dysfunction – how much sleep is impacting your daily life

Scores on the PSQI range from 0 to 21, and anything less than five is indicative of some severe sleep difficulties.

We can already see by this brief description of the PSQI where Ralph might be having some problems – he usually can get to sleep just fine, so sleep latency is not his problem. What is concerning for Ralph is his sleep duration and his daytime dysfunction. It is interesting about his sleep efficiency – he usually wakes up in the very early morning, and sometimes he stays in bed trying unsuccessfully to get back to sleep. On those days, his sleep efficiency plummets. However, when he starts giving up on sleeping past these early hours, he gets up and does things, like spy on his neighbors. When he does this, his sleep efficiency technically increases. Either way, Ralph is scoring low on the PSQI due to his extremely low sleep duration, occasionally low sleep efficiency, his daytime dysfunction, and the fact that he is subjectively miserable with his sleep quality.

This could be highly problematic for Ralph. Subjectively, it already is – despite getting up and doing what he has to do, Ralph is desperate for a good night sleep, and thinking about sleep occupies most of his waking hours. Evidence-wise, a lower PSQI score is associated with a wide assortment of negative health and well-being outcomes. Using items from the PSQI, researchers have found that lower sleep duration is associated with a significantly increased chance of getting the common cold when being experimentally exposed to the virus[7] (Cohen et al., 2009). Lower PSQI scores are associated with lung disease exacerbations (Shorofsky et al., 2019), vertigo (Du et al., 2023), poorer cognitive functioning, anxiety, depression (Gadie et al., 2017), and pain conditions (Afolalu et al., 2018), just to name a few. Ralph really needs to fix his sleep!

While we can't use his PSQI score alone to diagnose him with insomnia, there is quite a lot of research showing a high correlation between PSQI scores and an insomnia diagnosis (e.g., Backhaus et al., 2002; Mollayeva, 2016; Tsai et al., 2005). Despite his PSQI score, we still need a more formal diagnosis if we are going to help Ralph (and to justify the name of this book) – so let's move on to defining insomnia.

Ralph's Diagnosis – Insomnia?

Ralph is never officially given an insomnia diagnosis by someone trained to do so, but we have some good guidelines to follow to see if his symptoms would have warranted the diagnosis. Since there are no blood tests, or brain scans, or other techniques that we can use to say someone has insomnia and most other mental illnesses, we must rely on evidence-based guidelines put forth by the professionals. In order to standardize approaches to diagnosing and treating mental health disorders, the American Psychiatric Association developed the Diagnostic and Statistical Manual of Mental Disorders, known as the DSM. The DSM is currently in

Table 9.1 DSM-5 Diagnostic Criteria for Insomnia Disorder as Endorsed by Ralph Roberts

Criteria	*Criteria Description*	*Endorsed by Ralph Roberts?*
A	The chief complaint of the person is that they are dissatisfied with either how much sleep they are getting or the quality of the sleep they are getting. This complaint must be associated with one or more of the following:	Yes
	1 Person cannot fall asleep when they want to start sleeping (sleep initiation)	No
	2 Once they do fall asleep, they cannot stay asleep – that is, they wake up frequently during the night, or if they wake up during the night, they can't get back to sleep	Yes
	3 They wake up much earlier in the morning than intended, and cannot go back to sleep	Yes
B	The problems they are experiencing in Criteriona A are causing them significant distress. It causes them problems with their social life, or with their jobs, school, or other parts of life that are important to them	Yes
C	The problem they report in criterion A occurs at least three nights of the week	Yes
D	The problem has been happening for at least three months	Yes
E	The sleep problems occur, even though there is plenty of opportunity for the person to sleep	Yes
F	The insomnia they are experiencing is not better explained by another disorder like narcolepsy, sleep apnea, and so forth.	Yes
G	The insomnia is not due to the use of a medication or other substance	Yes
H	A mental disorder or other medical disorder does not explain what is experienced in criterion A	Yes

its fifth Edition (DSM-5, American Psychiatric Association, 2013), and it is used for evidence-based diagnosing in research, clinical care, and insurance practices. It has its problems, but it is the way most of us know what we are referring to when someone is diagnosed with a disorder, such as insomnia. Let's look at the DSM-5 criteria for insomnia disorder and see if the diagnosis Ralph gives himself is correct (see Table 9.1).

In order to be diagnosed with insomnia, the patient must meet all criteria, which Ralph certainly does. However, the most important criterion is the first one – the person must be dissatisfied with their sleep. If someone is not sleeping and has no problems with this, then it is not technically a disorder.[8] Ralph does have a problem with this, so let's review all the criteria.

Ralph is dissatisfied with his sleep, and the dissatisfaction comes from the fact that he wakes up after he has fallen asleep and then cannot get back to sleep. We call this Wake After Sleep Onset. Now, I said yes to both numbers 2 and 3 on this, because I think at the beginning of Ralph's sleep problems, when he was waking up at 4 or 5 in the morning, it was just a problem of waking up too early. As we progress in the novel, he starts waking up at 3, then 2, etc., which meets more of the second part of criterion A. Based on where his sleep ends up, I would say he has sleep maintenance insomnia – he is awake for long periods of time after he has initially fallen asleep.

Criterion B is met, and Ralph is constantly in a state of distress as he tries to navigate the world on a very short amount of sleep. His lack of sleep causes him to be short with Bill, forget to get groceries, and see small bald men and mystical auras. Sounds pretty intense! For Criteria C and D, this has been occurring every night for the last six months, so there is no problem meeting these criteria. As a retired individual, Ralph definitely meets Criterion E – he has plenty of time to sleep, which is something that makes his sleep problems even more daunting to him. For criteria F, G, and H, besides the sleep problems, Ralph is an extremely healthy 70-year-old. He has no other health conditions, and he takes no medications that would better explain his sleep problems.

In the end, Ralph would probably receive the following diagnosis – Insomnia disorder, persistent (symptoms have lasted more than three months), of the sleep maintenance type. This is lucky for Stephen King – how embarrassing if he had gotten the diagnosis wrong in the title!

If Ralph had gone to a sleep clinic, or even to his primary care physician, and received the diagnosis, there would have been several treatments available to him. From the biomedical perspective, he may have been prescribed medications such as zolpidem (e.g. Ambien) or temazepam (e.g. Restoril). Both are sedative hypnotics and should only be used in the short term, as they can have some significant side effects and can also lead to dependency.

He may have been prescribed those just so he can finally get some sleep, but then other treatments would need to be pursued. Luckily, on the biopsychosocial side of the coin, we have the gold standard for insomnia treatment – Cognitive Behavioral Therapy for Insomnia or CBT-I.

CBT to the Rescue!

Between the 1950s and the 1970s, a revolution happened that a lot of people aren't aware of – the cognitive revolution. In part, it was a reaction to the behaviorism that had dominated psychology earlier in the 20th century (Miller, 2003). Behaviorism was the idea that what mattered when it came to psychology, and who we are, was what was observable. Only that which could be seen was important, and what was important was gathered through learning – think of Pavlov's dogs or Skinner's use of reinforcement and punishment to train pigeons. The point was – everything was observable, and everything that we are is basically a learned reaction to our environment.

At some point, luckily, some psychologist and other scientists were like – "Hey – what about thinking? Isn't what we think important?" We can't observe it, but that doesn't mean it's not important. This is my very rudimentary explanation of the cognitive revolution. In this (re)newed inclusion of thoughts and beliefs in psychology emerged Aaron T Beck and cognitive therapy (Beck, 1970), later known as Cognitive Behavioral Therapy. The idea behind Beck's therapeutic approach was that distorted thinking patterns, such as overgeneralizations, jumping to conclusions, and catastrophizing, led to distress, maladaptive behavior, and depression. Later, the behavioral component was brought back in – CBT is now a therapeutic approach that emphasizes the interactions that occur between one's thoughts, feelings, and behavior.

Today, research has shown that CBT is one of the most effective forms of therapy – it has been shown to be highly effective for cannabis and nicotine dependence, anxiety, bulimia, and anger and aggression (Hofman et al., 2012). A specialized form of CBT that focuses solely on insomnia (CBT-I) has been shown to be extremely effective (Hertenstein et al., 2022; Mitchell et al., 2012; van der Zweerde et al., 2019).

There are four main parts to CBT-I: (1) Sleep Restriction Therapy, (2) Stimulus Control Therapy, (3) Sleep Hygiene, and (4) Cognitive Therapy (Walker et al., 2022). The first component, sleep restriction therapy, is, in a sense, focused on increasing sleep efficiency by having you spend less time in your bed. Depending on their sleep problems, patients get a prescribed bedtime and a prescribed wake time. This sleep restriction is monitored and modified as needed.

Stimulus control therapy focuses on reducing the other things around you that have been associated with your sleep attempts, for example, if you often read while trying to fall asleep, or watch TV, and so forth. The therapy involves getting patients to do the following: get into bed only when tired, use your bed for only sleeping and sex, if you can't sleep within 20 minutes, get out of the bed, and do this throughout the night if you need to (Walker et al., 2022).

Sleep hygiene is more of an educational component. It is about teaching people about how caffeine and alcohol can impact their sleep, the dangers of napping, the importance of creating a calm and cool sleeping environment, and the role exercise can play. The cognitive therapy aspect involves making sure that patients have realistic expectations for their sleep, that they challenge dysfunctional sleep-related thoughts, and then modify them to be more productive (Walker et al., 2022).

CBT-I occurs in about seven sessions. The first session is longest and can take up to 90 minutes as sleep is assessed, as well as a plethora of biopsychosocial factors impacting the person's sleep. After that, each session lasts about 30 minutes to an hour. In addition to attending sessions, patients will be asked to fill out a daily sleep diary.

This is our current gold standard treatment for insomnia, and as stated earlier, multiple systematic reviews and meta-analyses have found it highly effective. If Ralph had gone to the doctor and was referred to a CBT-I therapist, some of his issues might have been resolved (except for those pesky small bald guys). But Ralph never did go to a doctor or seek professional help. Why?

Not Seeking Care

> He wasn't going to call Litchfield back. Period.
>
> (King, 2016, p.58)

Lichfield is Dr. Litchfield – Ralph and Carolyn's family doctor. Dr. Litchfield is thoroughly entrenched in the biomedical model. Sick? Take some medicine. As Joe Wyzer states: "he's a nice enough guy, but he loves that prescription pad" (King, 2016, p.140). He is also fully entrenched in gender bias when it comes to treating his patients. When Carolyn starts suffering from severe headaches, she visits Dr. Litchfield to determine what is wrong. Without much of an investigation, Dr. Litchfield states it is simply tension headaches and prescribes some extra-strength Tylenol. This follows a long line of gendered thinking in health care, where it is assumed that women are more pain-averse and that they are more willing to report pain (Samulowitz et al., 2018). This same review found that health care providers were more likely to see women experiencing pain as emotional, complaining, and making up the pain. Much of this stemmed from providers believing that what the women were experiencing was all in their heads.

Turns out it was all in her head, but in the form of a brain tumor. This misdiagnosis leads to Ralph's mistrust of medical providers, and in particular Litchfield. Negative experiences often lead to medical mistrust, which then leads to avoidance of care and lower use of medical services (Benkert et al., 2019; Shukla et al., 2025). Another important factor in patients choosing providers is the physician's communication style. When a provider doesn't seem to listen to the patient, they are much less likely to use that provider (Victoor et al., 2012). Not surprisingly, when the provider has a low caring style, patients are less satisfied (Cousin et al., 2012). The result is that Ralph cancels his appointment with Dr. Litchfield and relies instead on the folk remedies and alternative medicine suggestions of those around him (see Box 9.3 for more on who is helping him with his insomnia).

Box 9.3 The Importance of Ralph's Weak Ties

We talked about all the folk and alternative remedies that were given to Ralph to help cure his insomnia, but we didn't talk too much about WHO was supplying those suggestions. This brings up an important topic in health psychology – the so called "weak" social ties. If you think back to our conversation on social integration (SI) in Chapter 5, you will remember that we named eight social roles that were important for health: spouse, parent. other relative, friend, church member, volunteer, and employee. Yet when it comes to Ralph, he is fulfilling none of these social roles with the people who provide him with advice – with the exception of Bill McGovern, who would fit in the friend category, the rest would be considered acquaintances.

It turns out that acquaintances are important too. Granovetter (1973) called these weak ties – relationships you have with people around you that are not intimate, that do not involve high arousal of emotion, and that do occur with any frequency. Studies conducted by Sandstrom and Dunn (2014) found students that had interactions with classmates considered acquaintances showed greater happiness and sense of belonging. This extended beyond the classroom to all of their daily weak tie interactions.

In a recent review of the weak ties literature, Moreton and colleagues (2023) found that weak ties are frequent and could be great potential sources of support – and indeed most people view them as supportive. Most importantly for Ralph, weak ties are often the source of useful information. Since you have a lot more weak ties to draw on than strong ones, you have a better chance of finding a weak tie with information related to your problem or condition.

Ralph's weak ties provide him with a lot of support and information (Mike Hanlon, from *It*, is the librarian who leads him to all the books on sleep). Even if none of that information helped him, at least he learned about the joys of honeycomb.

Folk Remedies and Alternative Medicine

Prior to seeking out the over-the-counter remedies at the Rite-Aid, Ralph tries an exhaustive list of what many of us would call folk remedies – the tips and tricks for treating our ills that get passed down from generation to generation. While Ralph is weary of conventional medicine, he is willing to give the folk remedies a try, and then the alternative medicine approaches[9] suggested by Joe Wyzer. As we discussed in Chapter 2, health psychology is evidence-based. The question we must ask ourselves here is: even though they didn't work for Ralph, is there any evidence that the folk remedies and alternative medicine suggestions he was given work?

> "Whiskey is the answer" – Bill McGovern
>
> (King, 2016, p.56)

One of the first folk remedies suggested to Ralph is by his downstairs neighbor, Bill McGovern. Bill states that all Ralph needs to do is down a half shot of whiskey with honey about 15 minutes before he wants to go to sleep. Bill's evidence for the efficacy of this treatment? It worked for him. Of course, in health psychology, anecdotal evidence, or evidence from a subject pool of one, does not make an evidence-based practice, so what does the research say about this intervention?

For people who do not have a substance use disorder, like Ralph Roberts, alcohol does hasten the time it takes to fall asleep (Thakkar et al., 2015). Chances are that when Bill was describing his insomnia, he had the sleep-onset variety (trouble falling asleep). Thus, he became one of the numerous people out there who use alcohol somewhat successfully to usher in sleep (Roehrs & Roth, 2001). However, alcohol does not have the ability to keep you asleep. Which makes this a counter-intuitive treatment for Ralph, who has no problem falling asleep, but can't seem to get back to sleep once he wakes up later in the night. Alcohol increases the time you spend in NREM sleep, that sleep you experience more in the beginning of your sleep cycle, but it seriously suppresses your REM sleep. Conclusion – even though that half shot of whiskey might have helped Bill fall asleep, it probably disrupted his sleep later in the night – exactly what Ralph does not want.

> "Little piece of honeycomb just before bedtime" – John Leydecker
> (King, 2016, p.123)

But what about the honey aspect of Bill's remedy – what is that about? Bill's isn't the only advice involving honey. After Ralph gives a statement to the police regarding Ed Deepneu's violence against his wife, Detective John Leydecker offers his sage insomnia advice – honeycomb. All Ralph needs to do, Leydecker insists, is ingest the honey, chew and spit out the waxy comb, and he will be asleep in no time.

One reason honey may be seen as a good sleep remedy is its ability to suppress coughs, especially in children (Cohen et al., 2012). Since having a cough may keep people awake at night, the ability of honey to stop it may have created this sleep-honey association. However, the jury is still out on whether honey is the best cough-suppressant or upper respiratory illness treatment (Abuelgasim et al., 2021; Kuitunen & Renko, 2023), so we can't hop on the honey bandwagon yet. Since we don't have a clear understanding of the effectiveness of honey for cough, and Ralph's insomnia wasn't a result of an upper respiratory tract infection anyway, this was probably not the advice he needed for insomnia. And while Ralph found no improvement in his sleep, he did find some improvement in his mood – he really enjoyed that honeycomb!

> "That cammy's a beaut" – Trigger Vachon
> (King, 2016, p.124)

One recommendation made to Ralph is chamomile tea. Trigger Vachon, driver for Derry Drycleaners and an acquaintance of Ralph, swears by the herbal remedy. Unfortunately, the evidence for its effectiveness is mixed. One recent review and meta-analysis on the use of chamomile found that when they aggregated the results of ten RCTs, they found that chamomile was effective for reducing the number of times one awakens during the night, but it had no impact on how long someone slept or how efficient their sleep was (Kazemi et al., 2024).

> "Give these guys a try" – Joe Wyzer
>
> (King, 2016, p.143)

Finally, Ralph gives up on the folk remedies and heads to the pharmacy for some over-the-counter relief. Luckily, he runs into the pharmacist Joe Wyzer, who offers some different suggestions. The guys that Joe Wyzer is referring to are an acupuncturist and a hypnotist. Both acupuncture and hypnosis would be considered alternative medicine treatments as opposed to folk remedies, so we have a bit more data regarding their effectiveness.

Let's start with acupuncture, which is a Traditional Chinese Medicine (TCM) treatment. The idea here is that your body's organs do not work in isolation; they are all interconnected and seeking balance. Acupuncture involves placing acupuncture needles on certain points of the body that are believed to be key points of flow and balance (Huang et al., 2009). The evidence here is mixed, as acupuncture studies are often missing a key component – a placebo arm (head back to Chapter 4 for the importance of placebos in clinical research). Without this placebo arm, it is hard to say how much of the insomnia benefits are from the actual acupuncture versus the expectancy placebo effect. Nevertheless, there seem to be some promising findings – with acupuncture showing positive effects on sleep latency, sleep efficiency, sleep duration, and sleep quality (Huang et al., 2009; Shergis et al., 2016). Chances are, if Ralph hadn't been struck by another kind of sharp item, the acupuncture might have helped. Even if it was "just" a placebo effect, I am sure he would have been grateful for any help he could get.

The results for hypnosis don't look as promising. For hypnosis, we do have randomized controlled trials that we can look at – where those receiving hypnosis are compared with a waitlist control as well as a sham treatment. Hypnosis was found to improve the length of sleep latency when compared to the waitlist condition, but no differences were found compared to sham treatment (Lam et al., 2015). This suggests that any benefits from hypnosis are due to placebo effects as opposed to something specific about hypnosis. A more recent review found inconclusive results (Mamoune et al., 2022). It seems like Joe Wyzer was a bit off with this recommendation – but no worries, what Ralph actually needed was a showdown with a small psychotic bald man in another dimension to cure his insomnia. No way for a Rite-Aid pharmacist to have known that!

Conclusion

For those who have suffered from it, insomnia can truly be a horror of an experience. That makes it the perfect disorder for Stephen King to sink his teeth into. I hope that this chapter has given you some insight into your own sleep, so that you can now go and sink your own teeth into a good night's rest!

Versions of *Insomnia*

Novel: King, S. (1994). *Insomnia*. Viking Press.
Audiobook (Audible Edition)[10]: King, S. (1994). *Insomnia* (E. Wallach, Narr.) [Audiobook]. Simon & Schuster Audio.

Learn More Questions

1 Find the original PSQI article by Buysse and colleagues (1989) and fill it out for Ralph Roberts. Using their provided scoring instructions, what score does he get? Based on the article, what kinds of health and wellbeing outcomes might Ralph expect based on his score?
2 We discussed some of the folk remedies suggested to Ralph Roberts, but not all of them. For example, what about the lemon and hot water Mrs. Rapaport recommends? Seek out the peer-reviewed literature on the other remedies discussed in this book. Do they fare better evidence-wise than what was discussed in this chapter? What other folk remedies are out there for sleep problems, and are they backed by any evidence beyond the anecdotal?
3 At one point, Sue, the cashier at the Red Apple, purchases Ralph a Magic Eye that he can hang around his neck. Think about what was discussed in Chapter 4 about placebos and voodoo curses. How do you think this amulet will help Ralph's insomnia?

Notes

1 Though one study demonstrated the timing of the circadian rhythm is about six minutes shorter for women than for men (Duffy et al., 2011). No wonder it never feels like there is enough hours in the day!
2 Pittsburgh to the rescue – again!
3 As described in Chapter 8, actigraphy is measured using a watch-like device that calculates movement to estimate sleep.
4 Could be indicative of sleep apnea, a problem impacting the airway muscles during sleep.
5 Could be indicative of restless legs syndrome, a movement disorder where there are uncomfortable sensations cause the urge to move the legs.
6 This is indicative of one of the parasomnias – disorders that involve abnormal behaviors, feelings and perceptions during sleep.
7 For more on these common cold studies, see Chapter 8.
8 This always makes me think of the quote attributed to Edith Piaf, the famous French singer: "For me, sleep is a waste of time. I'm afraid to sleep. It's a form of death." While she would never have gone to get an insomnia diagnosis because of her sleeping, it doesn't mean her health wouldn't suffer because of the lack of sleep. In fact, she died at 47 due to liver cancer, while also having many other contributing health problems.
9 Alternative medicine is different from folk remedies in that it is a bit more systematic. These are health practices that have standard forms of training and delivery (think acupuncture, hypnosis, and so forth) but are most often not part of traditional medical school training and are not part of health insurance coverage. Though this is changing!
10 I really enjoyed Eli Wallach's reading of *Insomnia*. Many people complain about the sound effects in these reading, but I think the mastery of Wallach's narration makes up for it.

Bibliography

Abuelgasim, H., Albury, C., & Lee, J. (2021). Effectiveness of honey for symptomatic relief in upper respiratory tract infections: A systematic review and meta-analysis. *BMJ Evidence-Based Medicine*, *26*(2), 57–64. https://doi.org/10.1136/bmjebm-2020-111336

Afolalu, E. F., Ramlee, F., & Tang, N. K. (2018). Effects of sleep changes on pain-related health outcomes in the general population: A systematic review of longitudinal studies with exploratory meta-analysis. *Sleep Medicine Reviews*, *39*, 82–97. https://doi.org/10.1016/j.smrv.2017.08.001

American Psychiatric Association. (2013). *Diagnostic and statistical manual of mental disorders* (5th ed.). https://doi.org/10.1176/appi.books.9780890425596

Azizi-Zeinalhajlou, A., Mirghafourvand, M., Nadrian, H., Samei Sis, S., & Matlabi, H. (2022). The contribution of social isolation and loneliness to sleep disturbances among older adults: A systematic review. *Sleep and Biological Rhythms*, *20*(2), 153–163. https://doi.org/10.1007/s41105-022-00380-x

Backhaus, J., Junghanns, K., Broocks, A., Riemann, D., & Hohagen, F. (2002). Test–retest reliability and validity of the Pittsburgh Sleep Quality Index in primary insomnia. *Journal of Psychosomatic Research*, *53*(3), 737–740. https://doi.org/10.1016/S0022-3999(02)00330-6

Beck, A. T. (1970). Cognitive therapy: Nature and relation to behavior therapy. *Behavior Therapy*, *1*(2), 184–200.

Benkert, R., Cuevas, A., Thompson, H. S., Dove-Medows, E., & Knuckles, D. (2019). Ubiquitous yet unclear: A systematic review of medical mistrust. *Behavioral Medicine*, *45*(2), 86–101. https://doi.org/10.1080/08964289.2019.1588220

Buysse, D. J., Reynolds III, C. F., Monk, T. H., Berman, S. R., & Kupfer, D. J. (1989). The Pittsburgh Sleep Quality Index: A new instrument for psychiatric practice and research. *Psychiatry Research*, *28*(2), 193–213.

Cohen, H. A., Rozen, J., Kristal, H., Laks, Y., Berkovitch, M., Uziel, Y., … & Efrat, H. (2012). Effect of honey on nocturnal cough and sleep quality: A double-blind, randomized, placebo-controlled study. *Pediatrics*, *130*(3), 465–471. https://doi.org/10.1542/peds.2011-3075

Cohen, S., Doyle, W. J., Alper, C. M., Janicki-Deverts, D., & Turner, R. B. (2009). Sleep habits and susceptibility to the common cold. *Archives of Internal Medicine*, *169*(1), 62–67. https://doi.org/10.1001/archinternmed.2008.505

Cousin, G., Mast, M. S., Roter, D. L., & Hall, J. A. (2012). Concordance between physician communication style and patient attitudes predicts patient satisfaction. *Patient Education and Counseling*, *87*(2), 193–197. https://doi.org/10.1016/j.pec.2011.08.004

de Feijter, M., O'connor, M. F., Arizmendi, B. J., Ikram, M. A., & Luik, A. I. (2021). The longitudinal association of actigraphy-estimated sleep with grief in middle-aged and elderly persons. *Journal of Psychiatric Research*, *137*, 66–72. https://doi.org/10.1016/j.jpsychires.2021.02.042

Deng, M., Qian, M., Lv, J., Guo, C., & Yu, M. (2023). The association between loneliness and sleep quality among older adults: A systematic review and meta-analysis. *Geriatric Nursing*, *49*, 94–100. https://doi.org/10.1016/j.gerinurse.2022.11.013

Du, Z., Wang, G., Yan, D., Yang, F., & Bing, D. (2023). Relationships between the Pittsburgh Sleep Quality Index (PSQI) and vertigo outcome. *Neurological Research*, *45*(4), 291–299. https://doi.org/10.1080/01616412.2022.2132728

Duda, M., Domagalik, A., Orlowska-Feuer, P., Krzysztynska-Kuleta, O., Beldzik, E., Smyk, M. K., … & Sarna, T. (2020). Melanopsin: From a small molecule to brain functions. *Neuroscience & Biobehavioral Reviews*, *113*, 190–203. https://doi.org/10.1016/j.neubiorev.2020.03.012

Duffy, J. F., Cain, S. W., Chang, A. M., Phillips, A. J., Münch, M. Y., Gronfier, C., … & Czeisler, C. A. (2011). Sex difference in the near-24-hour intrinsic period of the human circadian timing system. *Proceedings of the National Academy of Sciences*, *108*(supplement_3), 15602–15608. https://doi.org/10.1073/pnas.1010666108

Duffy, J. F., Zitting, K. M., & Chinoy, E. D. (2015). Aging and circadian rhythms. *Sleep Medicine Clinics*, *10*(4), 423. https://doi.org/10.1016/j.jsmc.2015.08.002

Gadie, A., Shafto, M., Leng, Y., & Kievit, R. A. (2017). How are age-related differences in sleep quality associated with health outcomes? An epidemiological investigation in a UK cohort of 2406 adults. *BMJ Open*, *7*(7), e014920.

Grandner, M. A. (2016). Sleep, health, and society. *Sleep Medicine Clinics*, *12*(1), 1. https://doi.org/10.1016/j.jsmc.2016.10.012

Granovetter, M. S. (1973). The strength of weak ties. *American Journal of Sociology*, *78*(6), 1360–1380.

Hertenstein, E., Trinca, E., Wunderlin, M., Schneider, C. L., Zuest, M. A., Feher, K. D., … & Nissen, C. (2022). Cognitive behavioral therapy for insomnia in patients with mental disorders and comorbid insomnia: A systematic review and meta-analysis. *Sleep Medicine Reviews*, *62*, 101597. https://doi.org/10.1016/j.smrv.2022.101597

Hirshkowitz, M., Whiton, K., Albert, S. M., Alessi, C., Bruni, O., DonCarlos, L., … & Ware, J. C. (2015). National Sleep Foundation's updated sleep duration recommendations. *Sleep Health*, *1*(4), 233–243. https://doi.org/10.1016/j.sleh.2015.10.004

Hofmann, S. G., Asnaani, A., Vonk, I. J., Sawyer, A. T., & Fang, A. (2012). The efficacy of cognitive behavioral therapy: A review of meta-analyses. *Cognitive Therapy and Research*, *36*(5), 427–440. https://doi.org/10.1007/s10608-012-9476-1

Hood, S., & Amir, S. (2017). The aging clock: Circadian rhythms and later life. *The Journal of Clinical Investigation*, *127*(2), 437–446. https://doi.org/10.1172/JCI90328

Huang, W., Kutner, N., & Bliwise, D. L. (2009). A systematic review of the effects of acupuncture in treating insomnia. *Sleep Medicine Reviews*, *13*(1), 73–104. https://doi.org/10.1016/j.smrv.2008.04.002

Kazemi, A., Shojaei-Zarghani, S., Eskandarzadeh, P., & Hashempur, M. H. (2024). Effects of chamomile (Matricaria chamomilla L.) on sleep: A systematic review and meta-analysis of clinical trials. *Complementary Therapies in Medicine*, *84*, 103071 https://doi.org/10.1016/j.ctim.2024.103071

King, S. (2016). *Insomnia*. Scribner. https://www.amazon.com/dp/B00P42WROG

Kuitunen, I., & Renko, M. (2023). Honey for acute cough in children—A systematic review. *European Journal of Pediatrics*, *182*(9), 3949–3956. https://doi.org/10.1007/s00431-023-05066-1

Lam, T. H., Chung, K. F., Yeung, W. F., Yu, B. Y. M., Yung, K. P., & Ng, T. H. Y. (2015). Hypnotherapy for insomnia: A systematic review and meta-analysis of randomized controlled trials. *Complementary Therapies in Medicine*, *23*(5), 719–732. https://doi.org/10.1016/j.ctim.2015.07.011

Lancel, M., Stroebe, M., & Eisma, M. C. (2020). Sleep disturbances in bereavement: A systematic review. *Sleep Medicine Reviews*, *53*, 101331. https://doi.org/10.1016/j.smrv.2020.101331

Li, J., Vitiello, M. V., & Gooneratne, N. S. (2022). Sleep in normal aging. *Sleep Medicine Clinics*, *17*(2), 161–171. https://doi.org/10.1016/j.jsmc.2022.02.007

Mamoune, S., Mener, E., Chapron, A., & Poimboeuf, J. (2022). Hypnotherapy and insomnia: A narrative review of the literature. *Complementary Therapies in Medicine*, *65*, 102805. https://doi.org/10.1016/j.ctim.2022.102805

Meyer, N., Harvey, A. G., Lockley, S. W., & Dijk, D. J. (2022). Circadian rhythms and disorders of the timing of sleep. *The Lancet*, *400*(10357), 1061–1078. https://doi.org/10.1016/S0140-6736(22)00877-7

Milic, J., Saavedra Perez, H., Zuurbier, L. A., Boelen, P. A., Rietjens, J. A., Hofman, A., & Tiemeier, H. (2019). The longitudinal and cross-sectional associations of grief and complicated grief with sleep quality in older adults. *Behavioral Sleep Medicine*, *17*(1), 31–40. https://doi.org/10.1080/15402002.2016.1276016

Miller, G. A. (2003). The cognitive revolution: A historical perspective. *Trends in Cognitive Sciences*, *7*(3), 141–144. https://doi.org/10.1016/S1364-6613(03)00029-9

Miner, B., & Kryger, M. H. (2016). Sleep in the aging population. *Sleep Medicine Clinics*, *12*(1), 31. https://doi.org/10.1016/j.jsmc.2016.10.008

Mitchell, M. D., Gehrman, P., Perlis, M., & Umscheid, C. A. (2012). Comparative effectiveness of cognitive behavioral therapy for insomnia: A systematic review. *BMC Family Practice*, *13*(1), 40. https://www.biomedcentral.com/1471-2296/13/40

Mollayeva, T., Thurairajah, P., Burton, K., Mollayeva, S., Shapiro, C. M., & Colantonio, A. (2016). The Pittsburgh sleep quality index as a screening tool for sleep dysfunction in clinical and non-clinical samples: A systematic review and meta-analysis. *Sleep Medicine Reviews*, *25*, 52–73. https://doi.org/10.1016/0165-1781(89)90047-4

Moreton, J., Kelly, C. S., & Sandstrom, G. M. (2023). Social support from weak ties: Insight from the literature on minimal social interactions. *Social and Personality Psychology Compass*, *17*(3), e12729. https://doi.org/10.1111/spc3.12729

Patton, A. P., & Hastings, M. H. (2018). The suprachiasmatic nucleus. *Current Biology*, *28*(15), R816–R822. https://doi.org/10.1016/j.cub.2018.06.052

Roehrs, T., & Roth, T. (2001). Sleep, sleepiness, and alcohol use. *Alcohol Research & Health*, *25*(2), 101–109.

Samulowitz, A., Gremyr, I., Eriksson, E., & Hensing, G. (2018). "Brave men" and "emotional women": A theory-guided literature review on gender bias in health care and gendered norms towards patients with chronic pain. *Pain Research and Management*, *2018*(1), 6358624. https://doi.org/10.1155/2018/6358624

Sandstrom, G. M., & Dunn, E. W. (2014). Social interactions and well-being: The surprising power of weak ties. *Personality and Social Psychology Bulletin*, *40*(7), 910–922. https://doi.org/10.1177/0146167214529799

Shear, M. K. (2015). Complicated grief. *New England Journal of Medicine*, *372*(2), 153–160. https://doi.org/10.1056/NEJMcp1315618

Shergis, J. L., Ni, X., Jackson, M. L., Zhang, A. L., Guo, X., Li, Y., … & Xue, C. C. (2016). A systematic review of acupuncture for sleep quality in people with insomnia. *Complementary Therapies in Medicine*, *26*, 11–20. https://doi.org/10.1016/j.ctim.2016.02.007

Shorofsky, M., Bourbeau, J., Kimoff, J., Jen, R., Malhotra, A., Ayas, N., … & Canadian Respiratory Research Network. (2019). Impaired sleep quality in COPD is associated with exacerbations: The CanCOLD cohort study. *Chest*, *156*(5), 852–863. https://doi.org/10.1016/j.chest.2019.04.132

Shukla, M., Schilt-Solberg, M., & Gibson-Scipio, W. (2025). Medical mistrust: A concept analysis. *Nursing Reports*, *15*(3), 103. https://doi.org/10.3390/nursrep15030103

Stalder, T., Oster, H., Abelson, J. L., Huthsteiner, K., Klucken, T., & Clow, A. (2025). The cortisol awakening response: Regulation and functional significance. *Endocrine Reviews*, *46*(1), 43–59. https://doi.org/10.1210/endrev/bnae024

Thakkar, M. M., Sharma, R., & Sahota, P. (2015). Alcohol disrupts sleep homeostasis. *Alcohol*, *49*(4), 299–310. https://doi.org/10.1016/j.alcohol.2014.07.019Get rights and content

Tsai, P. S., Wang, S. Y., Wang, M. Y., Su, C. T., Yang, T. T., Huang, C. J., & Fang, S. C. (2005). Psychometric evaluation of the Chinese version of the Pittsburgh Sleep Quality Index (CPSQI) in primary insomnia and control subjects. *Quality of Life Research, 14*(8), 1943–1952. https://doi.org/10.1007/s11136-005-4346-x

van der Zweerde, T., Bisdounis, L., Kyle, S. D., Lancee, J., & van Straten, A. (2019). Cognitive behavioral therapy for insomnia: A meta-analysis of long-term effects in controlled studies. *Sleep Medicine Reviews, 48,* 101208. https://doi.org/10.1016/j.smrv.2019.08.002

Victoor, A., Delnoij, D. M., Friele, R. D., & Rademakers, J. J. (2012). Determinants of patient choice of healthcare providers: A scoping review. *BMC Health Services Research, 12*(1), 272. https://www.biomedcentral.com/1472-6963/12/272

Walker, J., Muench, A., Perlis, M. L., & Vargas, I. (2022). Cognitive Behavioral Therapy for Insomnia (CBT-I): A primer. *Klinicheskaia i spetsial'naia psikhologiia = Clinical Psychology and Special Education, 11*(2), 123–137. https://doi.org/10.17759/cpse.2022110208

10 The Horror of Behavior Change

At the end of the day, the ultimate goal of health psychology is to improve people's health. As stated in the mission of Division 38 (Society for Health Psychology) of the American Psychological Association:

"The Society for Health Psychology (SfHP) seeks to improve the lives of individuals and society by promoting health, preventing illness, and improving health care through research, practice, education, training, and advocacy." (Society for Health Psychology, 2023).

Think way back to the first chapter in this book, where we discussed how illness and death changed from infectious diseases to lifestyle diseases. One of the ways that health psychology seeks to improve people's health is through changing behaviors – getting people to eat better, exercise more, and quit health-compromising behaviors like smoking, excessive drinking, and risk-taking.

Stephen King used to be a pretty heavy cigarette smoker, so it is not hard to see where he may have come up with the idea for his short story *Quitters, Inc.* (see Box 10.1 for summary). The horror of it comes from how hard changing behaviors can be, especially ones that involve addictive substances like nicotine. Despite the challenge, health psychologists still seek better ways to make smoking cessation efforts easier and more successful – hopefully in better ways than *Quitters, Inc.*!

Box 10.1 ***Quitters, Inc.*** ⚠ **[Spoiler Alert]**

In 1978, Stephen King published a book of short stories called *Night Shift*. One of these stories, *Quitters, Inc.*, tells the story of Dick Morrison, and the horrifying lengths he will have to (need to) go to in order to quit smoking.

On a fateful business trip, Dick is at the airport when he runs into an old college buddy, Jimmy McCann. Both men are middle-aged, but it seems that Jimmy is looking much younger and healthier than Dick, and he also seems to be moving up the corporate ladder at a quicker pace.

Jimmy tells Dick that the key to his success – in terms of quitting smoking – is a company called Quitters, Inc. Jimmy claims that Quitters, Inc. has a miraculously high success rate –98% of their clients quit smoking,

DOI: 10.4324/9781003495994-10

and that they guarantee success. Jimmy leaves Dick with the card for Quitters, Inc. and tells him to consider it – as it has changed his life. Dick is a little unclear of what this company actually does as Jimmy signed a contract that included some sort of non-disclosure agreement. Jealous of Jimmy's success, but sensing something fishy in the method, the card goes in his pocket and out of his mind.

About a month after his run-in with Jimmy, Dick had left work early in order to drown his sorrows at a local bar. When he goes to pay his tab, the card he was given falls out of his pocket, and Quitters, Inc. makes a reappearance. Noticing the office is not too far away, Dick decides to take a stroll and see what Jimmy was on about. Observing the swankiness of the office building, Dick takes the elevator up to the office and gives his information to the receptionist. Shortly thereafter, he is seen by his appointed "counselor," Vic Donatti. Starting with the obvious "Do you want to quit smoking" question, Vic peppers Dick with a plethora of other questions, not all of them seeming to be related to the task at hand. Vic assures him that this is normal and that it is part of their "pragmatic" way of getting people to quit smoking. Vic then invites Dick back to the office the next day, when the treatment will begin.

Despite his reservations, especially considering he still does not know the nature of the treatment, Dick returns the next day. He is immediately told by Vic that his treatment has started. He assumes it will probably center around hypnosis or something similar, so he is taken aback when Vic shows him a rabbit being shocked when he tries to eat. It is explained that they can quickly and easily train the rabbit not to eat by shocking it, and that is how they will train Dick not to smoke. However, there is a caveat with the human no-smoking training – the person who will be shocked will not be Dick himself, but his wife.

Vic then explains that there is a hierarchy of "punishments" that will occur to his family and him every time he smokes a cigarette. The employees of Quitters, Inc. will be surveilling him constantly for the first month. The first time he smokes, his wife will be "the rabbit," the second time it will be his turn, the third time they both will be shocked, and the fourth time, it will be his developmentally disabled son. As more infractions occur, the severity of the punishments increases. Once he sees the nature of the treatment he is signed up for, he tries to back out but is informed by Vic that treatment has already begun.

While quitting is difficult, and he does slip, Dick is able to do it. However, he gains a bit of weight in the process, and soon weight loss becomes a goal within his Quitters, Inc. regime. He loses weight, quits smoking, is healthier than he has ever been, and even gets promoted at work. He himself then begins handing out Quitters, Inc. cards to others. Until a fateful day when he meets Jimmy again, looking even better than he did that day at the airport. He also meets Jimmy's wife, who gives Dick a glimpse at the price that was paid for Jimmy to get that way.

The Power of Smoking and Nicotine

In *Quitters, Inc.*, Dick's smoking is what we would call a health-compromising behavior. He has several other such behaviors, such as drinking and unhealthy eating, but let's focus on smoking. Smoking is one of the most dangerous of the health-compromising behaviors, accounting for a huge amount of preventable illness and death. It is also one of the hardest behaviors to change, and secondhand smoke can be just as dangerous to the people around the smoker as to the smoker themselves.[1]

Quitters, Inc. focuses on cigarette smoking, but let's discuss the substance within the cigarette that makes it so addictive – nicotine. When King published *Quitters, Inc.* in 1978, the rate of cigarette smoking in the US was almost 35% (American Lung Association, 2023). Today, that rate is about 11%. Despite the decrease in cigarette smoking, nicotine is still a very popular substance – it is just that the delivery system has changed. Now, instead of getting nicotine via a cigarette, people are using e-cigarettes, or vaping devices. For example, in the 18–25-year-old range, the rate of e-cig or vaping is around 25%.

The rise of e-cigarettes and vaping is an interesting story, given our topic of behavior change. Before I discuss what exactly nicotine is, how it works, and why it is so addictive, I want to delve into those number changes given above. It is fantastic that cigarette smoking has decreased so significantly since the 1960s and 1970s. If there is one behavior that we can easily point to and confidently say – that causes disease – it is cigarette smoking.

Why? Cigarettes don't just contain the nicotine that everyone wants, it contains thousands of other substances, many of which are toxic (Saha et al., 2007). Cigarette smoking accounts for 90% of all lung cancers and is responsible for one in four cardiovascular disease deaths (U.S. Department of Health and Human Services, 2014). Not to mention the increased risks cigarettes smoking poses to reproductive health, diabetes, and various other types of cancer.

Recognizing that it was the nicotine that was making it so hard for people to quit smoking, a man named Hon Lik created an e-cigarette device that allowed nicotine to be inhaled, but without those harmful tobacco byproducts (Razali, 2025). Inspired by his own father's lung cancer death, this device would be considered a harm-reduction technique – if we can't get people to quit nicotine, at least we can have them inhale it in a less toxic form. This way, they would not have to give up the physical sensation of smoking. E-cigarettes were also promoted as a smoking cessation tool – that they would help people "step down" to quitting cigarettes and nicotine altogether.

While the original motivation for e-cigarettes was for them only to be used by traditional cigarette smokers as a way to smoke more safely or quit the habit altogether, it unfortunately introduced a whole new population to nicotine. These are the younger generations we talked about – they have never smoked cigarettes – instead, they went straight to e-cigarettes and vaping. The American Lung Association (2023) reports that almost 5% of middle school students (11–14 years old) use e-cigarettes, and that about 2,200 children start smoking them every day. Some of you may be saying – well, at least that is better than smoking traditional cigarettes. Before you make that judgment, let's talk about that addictive substance that an 11-year-old might be breathing in, and what it might be doing to the mind and body. And then we can get to Quitters, Inc. – and the lengths people may need to go to in order to quit it!

Nicotine – It's a Hell of a Drug

> I think it was quitting smoking that slowed me down; nicotine is a great synapse enhancer. The problem, of course, is that it's killing you at the same time it's helping you compose.
>
> (King, 2020, p.153)

Here, Stephen King talks about the pace at which he writes. Famously, he has stated that he finished *The Running Man* (see Chapter 6) in a week. However, once he quit smoking, his speed writing days were numbered. That is because his several packs a day habit was delivering him a constant flow of nicotine – a pretty potent stimulant drug.

Stimulants are a class of drugs that increase activity within both the brain and body. You have your legal stimulants, like caffeine and nicotine, your prescription stimulants, like amphetamines used for attention deficit/hyperactivity disorder (ADHD), and your illicit stimulants like cocaine and methamphetamine. All of these substances work by communicating with specific receptors within the brain, to cause varying psychological sensations and physical changes. Let's see how this works with nicotine.

When nicotine is inhaled through the lungs, it enters your bloodstream almost immediately. Nicotine is one of the substances that can cross the blood–brain barrier, which is a layer of cells that prevents certain substances from entering the brain. Once it is through the barrier, it will bind to certain receptors in the brain called nicotinic acetylcholine receptors (Le Foll et al., 2022). The nicotine acts as an agonist here – that means it activates the receptor – leading to the release of dopamine, norepinephrine, and serotonin. These neurotransmitters increase heart rate, blood pressure, and attention, as well as feelings of pleasure. This can all happen within 30 seconds of that first inhale!

One of the problems with nicotine is the release of the neurotransmitter dopamine. Once nicotine has entered the brain, it very quickly makes changes to the neuronal circuitry – like activating dopaminergic neurons in two parts of the brain: the ventral tegmental area (VTA) and the nucleus accumbens (see Figure 10.1). The VTA and nucleus accumbens are part of the brain's reward system – this is why you get a quick and significant increase in pleasure with each puff. However, this reward system is also one of the reasons why it is so addictive.

Continuous use of nicotine will actually cause the brain to make some pretty significant changes, where it will become dependent on the nicotine to perform at the baseline level of mood and alertness. Many people will experience what we call tolerance, where they will need more and more of the substance to get the same

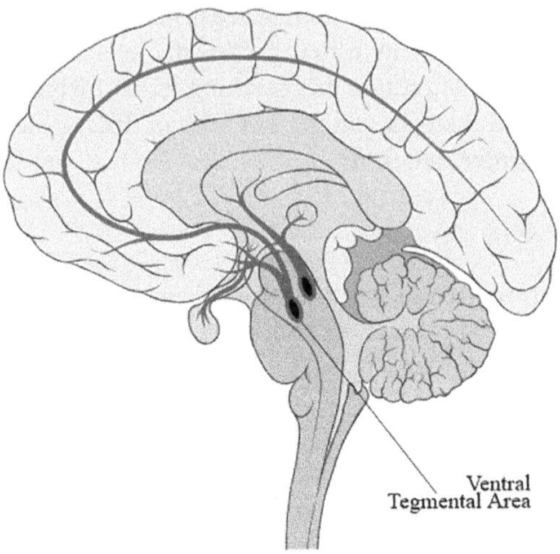

Figure 10.1 Location of Ventral Tegmental Area (VTA).

feelings of pleasure. This is where you may see someone smoking multiple packs a day to get the same effect that maybe just one or two cigarettes gave them in the past. Lastly, when people try to quit nicotine after prolonged and heavy use, these brain changes will lead to withdrawal symptoms. In the case of nicotine, without it, those dependent on it will experience the inability to concentrate, poor moods, anxiety, and weight gain. These extremely unpleasant and unwanted side effects that come with the initial withdrawal of nicotine from the system make quitting very difficult.

That is just a very brief summary of the biological mechanisms that make quitting smoking so hard. There are also psychological aspects to that habit that make it difficult. In the user's mind, smoking can be associated with pleasant things, especially if one has been smoking since their teenage years. You may associate it with "better times." Along these lines, it might be just something that you and a group of friends do together when you hang out, so it is indeed a pleasant social experience. To support this, research shows that smoking is "contagious," that is, you get it from your friend groups, and it is an important part of social network classification (Christakis & Fowler, 2008). It may also be an integral part of relaxation routines you have, from coffee breaks at work to smoking before bed. Being a smoker may also be an important part of one's self-identity. When they picture themselves, they may see a cigarette as an important accessory to who they are.

You can see all of this play out throughout Dick's behavior change journey. Many times, a reference is made to how "smug" non-smokers can be. It is unfair that they just cannot understand the actual physical changes caused by the addiction. Due to this lack of understanding, they can't do anything except assume quitting is easy. Dick is fully entrenched in this knowledge and his addiction – he knows as soon as he stubs out one of his cigs, he will be lighting up again in a few minutes. Even when he is in the waiting room of the company that specializes in getting people to quit smoking – he takes out a pack of cigarettes and looks for a non-existent ashtray. He starts imagining smoking a cigarette as soon as he gets out of there. As he has to wait, "his nicotine center was speaking quite loudly" (King, 2012, p.224).

But Quit You Must!

As health psychologists interested in getting people to improve their health, we do want people to quit nicotine, even when used in a "safer" form like e-cigarettes, lozenges, or patches. Why? In addition to changing various pathways in the brain, the stimulant nature of nicotine can harm other body systems – such as the cardiovascular system. For example, one study (Jolma et al., 2002) that looked at the effect of chewing nicotine gum found that the gum (when compared to placebo gum) caused significant increases in heart rate, blood pressure, and higher end-systolic wall stress (ESWS). ESWS is basically a measure of how much strain the wall of the heart ventricles is experiencing after it has ejected blood. This indicates that nicotine use is putting a lot of pressure on the heart and arteries.

Studies on e-cigarettes show this as well, and the American Heart Association (Wold et al., 2022) recently warned that even in younger e-cigarette users, they are seeing increases in the stiffness of artery walls and indications of oxidative stress. They also discuss recent findings regarding e-cigarettes' effect on the immune system, most notably an increase in inflammation. Nicotine can also cause insulin resistance, low-birth-weight babies, and changes in testosterone and estrogen that lead to a myriad of reproductive system issues (Tweed et al., 2012).

Regardless of its delivery system, nicotine is a highly addictive drug that significantly impacts people's health. Thus, it is incumbent on health psychologists to find a way to help people quit. The first challenge is to figure out how all of the factors mentioned here work together to keep people using, and how they can be used to raise awareness and change people's behavioral intentions – an indication of their level of motivation toward changing a health behavior, and how much effort they are willing to put into planning and making the change. There are two main behavior change theories we will talk about, especially in terms of Quitters, Inc. We have the Health Belief Model (HBM) and the Theory of Planned Behavior (TPB).

Health Belief Model

In their discussion at the airport, Jimmy illustrates perfectly what we call a "cue to action" in the HBM of Behavior Change. HBM was a theory of behavioral change that originated in the 1950s (Rosenstock, 1974) that focused on attitudes/cognitions people have around health behavior. The HBM states that the following are important cognitive constructs that must be considered when making health behavior change (see Figure 10.2):

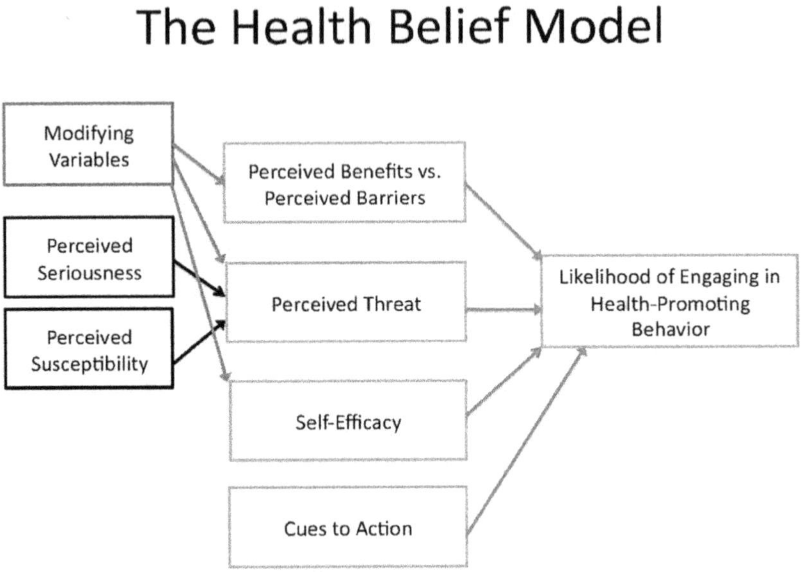

Figure 10.2 Schematic of the Health Belief Model.

The person's beliefs about a health threat. This consists of two things the person must perceive: (1) They are susceptible to a health problem (perceived susceptibility) and (2) that the health problem is severe (perceived severity).

The person's beliefs about the health behavior. This consists of (1) perceiving that changing the behavior will reduce the health threat (perceived benefits) and (2) that changing the behavior won't cause more problems than the health threat itself (perceived barriers).

In addition, newer formulations state that the person making the change must have self-efficacy – that is they must truly believe they have the capacity/ability to make the change. There is also included the idea of a cue to action – some sort of stimulus that causes the person to pursue behavior change.

Okay, now let's get back to Jimmy McCann. In the airport, he provides Dick with a pretty good narrative story about what prompted him to want to quit smoking. Let's look at it through the HBM:

Perceived susceptibility: Jimmy mentions several things that may have made him realize how susceptible he was to the health damage of cigarette smoking. One, his father has a heart attack, which may have brought his genetic susceptibility to the forefront. He is also told by his doctor that he has an ulcer.

Perceived severity: Not only did his dad have a heart attack, but he died from it, which increases Jimmy's knowledge of the severity of the health problems associated with smoking.

Perceived benefits: After giving him the ulcer diagnosis, Jimmy's doctor tells him that he needs to quit smoking – making for him the connection that quitting smoking will help relieve the ulcer. He is also told by his boss that he needs to get his act together, and Jimmy perceives quitting smoking as one way of getting that done.

Perceived barriers: While this part is not as explored in depth here, it may be because the barriers are quite intuitive – he is addicted to nicotine. All the things we mentioned above (dependency, tolerance, and withdrawal) are going to be put into the barriers category.

Self-efficacy: At first, Jimmy is missing this part of the puzzle. He struggles with his ability to quit and "was cheating like hell" until of course he is referred to Quitters, Inc. And while his marital problems, hacking cough, the death of his father, and so forth may have been an initial cue to action, I would make the argument that Quitters, Inc., when looked at through the HBM, offered the ultimate cue to action for Jimmy to change his behavior.

Quitters, Inc., in its unorthodox approach, addresses several aspects of HBM. The perceived susceptibility and severity were pretty much set – no more was needed here for Jimmy to want to make the change. I think it was the person's belief about the health behavior, the self-efficacy, and the cue to action that made the behavior change stick.

As stated above, the barriers to quitting smoking are clear, and biologically embedded, making it even more difficult to quit than heroin. In order to counter that, the perceived benefits of quitting have to significantly outweigh the barriers. That is exactly what Quitters, Inc. does – the benefits of quitting smoking are that you and your family members will not get severely shocked, beaten, or killed. A pretty convincing benefit!

As for the self-efficacy part – the wishy-washy feelings about being able to do it completely disappeared when family members' lives were threatened. If it were just a threat to his own safety and well-being, Jimmy may not have felt as capable. But since he is forced to be the protector, through his actions, he gains a certain amount of self-efficacy – his family's lives are completely within his control.

But perhaps the biggest thing that Quitters, Inc. provided was the cue to action. As soon as any client comes for the second appointment, the intervention starts right there and then. They have no choice – if they do not quit smoking immediately, really bad things are going to start happening.

Theory of Planned Behavior

HBM is not the only a theoretic model that has been developed to help inform and guide us in health change interventions. The TPB takes a slightly different view of people's attitudes toward behavior change (Ajzen, 1991). TPB is very concerned with how we form our behavioral intentions, and that it is our formed intentions

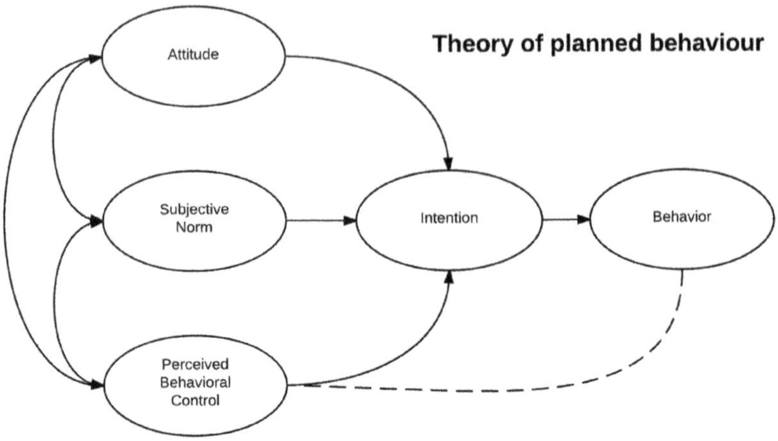

Figure 10.3 Schematic of the Theory of Planned Behavior.

that are going to lead to our behavior change. But what impacts our intentions? TPB says it is a combination of three factors (see Figure 10.3):

Attitudes: Our own personal attitudes toward the behavior and its effects
Subjective Norms: Beliefs that those around us have, and how much we care about their beliefs.
Perceived Control: Our belief in our ability to change

As you can see, attitudes and perceived control are very similar to the beliefs and self-efficacy aspects of HBM. What was not considered in HBM, though, was the subjective norm part – the idea that it is not just about our own attitudes and beliefs, but about those of the people around us.

This subjective norm aspect of deciding to make a behavioral change is described by both Jimmy McCann and Dick Morrison. When Jimmy describes his decision to quit smoking, he discusses the "pep talk" that his boss Bobby Crager gave him. In no uncertain terms, Jimmy is told that he needs to make some changes, or he will lose his job. This is the information that Jimmy needs to understand that the normative belief of his workspace is that he needs to change – and since he wants to keep his job, he does indeed care what this other person believes. According to the TPB, this will make him more likely to form an intention to quit, which he very much does.

⚠ **[Spoiler Alert]** We can also see this in Dick's behavior change journey, but this time, it is embodied by his wife, Cindy. In one of the (many) surprises in the book, Cindy does not seem to be as upset as we might expect her to be after she is kidnapped by Quitters, Inc. as a result of Dick having a drag of a cigarette while stuck in traffic. Despite being brought to the "rabbit room" against her will and being subjected to electrical shocks, she is on board with him quitting smoking, even if this is how it has to be done. The subjective norm here is that his wife is invested in him quitting and having a healthier lifestyle. Because he cares about Cindy and what she believes, he will continue to have the intention of not smoking. Even when the high-priced financial payment comes due – including a bill for the electricity they used to shock her – Cindy happily tells him to just pay it – as it is in service of him quitting smoking.

Now that we have a better understanding of how people get to the point of wanting to change – what are the techniques that are used to actually help them do it?

As we stated previously, nicotine is a highly addictive substance on the biological, psychological, and social levels. Planning interventions is difficult, and they have varying levels of success. Let's look at some of the ones that are alluded to or directly discussed in *Quitters, Inc.* Oddly enough, a lot of the intervention techniques I will be talking about are based on principles of behaviorism. We discussed this in Chapter 9 when we took a deep dive into the cognitive revolution. Behaviorism was all about what we learn, that we as humans are just made up of reactions to our environment, and what we learned from those reactions. To them, psychology is only what we can observe, and thinking doesn't really play a role. Aversion therapy and contingency contracting are based on the key tenets of behaviorism.

Aversion Therapy – Pavlov's Legacy

Before we discuss what is involved in aversion therapy, let us quickly go back to the late 1800s and discuss Ivan Pavlov. Much like Walter Cannon (Chapters 3 and 4), Pavlov was a physiologist who was interested in digestion. He performed a lot of his research on dogs, and it was through this that he unexpectedly developed the tenets of classical conditioning.

Salivation is an important part of digestion. It gets the food moist, making it easier to chew and swallow, and it also contains amylase that starts to break down components of food. Pavlov was studying this part of digestion when he noticed an odd phenomenon. When his research assistant brought in the dogs' food, they would start to salivate, indicating they were preparing to eat the meat in the bowls. That seems normal enough. What was not normal was that after a while, when the researcher would come into the room without the food, the dogs would still start to salivate (Eelen, 2018).

The idea here is that the dogs learned to associate the food with the research assistant, and due to these associations, they had a biological response. It doesn't have to be the happenstance sight and sound of research assistant entering a room – you can do some pairing – which is how Pavlov has become synonymous with ringing a bell and salivating. Here is how it works:

First, you have what we call the unconditioned stimulus (US) – this is what the food is in the scenario above – the food is the stimulus that naturally and automatically causes the dogs to salivate. That salivation to the food is what we call the unconditioned response (UR) – it is a completely natural and automatic biological response to the US.

We then have something that we call the neutral stimulus (NS) – something that on its own produces no natural and automatic response. Just a bell ringing on its own would not produce salivation in a dog – they don't want to eat a metal noise maker! But then the conditioning occurs – if I repeatedly pair the ringing bell with the food – the dog associates that metal noise maker with the food they want to eat. Suddenly, the ringing bell has become a conditioned stimulus (CS) – because when it is on its own (rings without food), it will now cause the dog to salivate, or the conditioned response (CR).

In summary, classical conditioning must have some sort of natural and automatic response that occurs with a certain stimulus. If you then pair that stimulus enough times with something that doesn't cause that automatic response initially, it eventually will. We discussed briefly in Chapter 2 about Stephen King's very early life – when he was in first grade and had to go to the ear doctor repeatedly to undergo excruciatingly painful eardrum piercing. He states that he remembers the smell in the doctor's office – that of the sterilizing rubbing alcohol. Before he went to these doctors' visits, he had no natural or automatic response to the rubbing alcohol – it was an NS for him. In that doctor's office, with that smell, he then experienced the ear procedure (the US) and the automatic pain response (the UR). Unfortunately, this happened several times, and King reports "that smell of alcohol, an aroma that still has the power to double my heartbeat in the space of five seconds." (King, 2020, p.25). Thus, the smell of rubbing alcohol became the CS, which elicits an automatic biological response (CR) stemming from the pain associated with it.

What does all this have to do with trying to get someone to stop smoking? The answer is aversion therapy – when we attempt to decrease the attractiveness of smoking by pairing it with something unpleasant (Hajek & Stead, 2001). One aversive therapy technique is called rapid smoking. This is equivalent to your parents putting you in a closet and forcing you to smoke a pack of cigarettes – in the hopes of you never wanting to smoke another one ever again. This is what Dick was referring to when he asked Jimmy if they "strap you down and make you smoke until you throw up?" (King, 2012, p.221).

Therapeutic-wise, rapid smoking involves making participants inhale from a cigarette every six to ten seconds (Hajek & Stead, 2001). They have to do this for a full three minutes, or until they are so sick they cannot smoke anymore. They then can take a break, but the procedure is repeated several times, and over several weeks. The participants focus on how bad cigarettes are making them feel, with the hope that they will become a CS for an unpleasant CR, and then they will want to quit being exposed to them.

As you might imagine, the approach has several flaws and is no longer used (at least by the medical professionals, I am not sure about parents!) The biggest problem was that there were high probabilities of nicotine poisoning and cardiac events. When you have that much of a stimulant in a short amount of time – your heart may not be able to handle it. Less severe versions have been attempted, but they don't seem to produce enough of an aversive effect to overcome the nicotine addiction.

Other aversive stimuli that have been tried are electrical shocks while smoking, snapping a rubber band on the wrist every time you smoke or want to smoke, and using a bitter substance in conjunction with smoking. Research, however, has shown that only rapid smoking works, but with only modest improvements, especially compared to the side effects (Hajek & Stead, 2001). Thus, this is rarely ever an option anymore (we will leave it for you to decide if this was a good or bad thing for Dick!).

Contingency Contracts – Skinner's Revenge

One thing that is still used today is contingency contracting, which is based on another behaviorism technique – operant conditioning. Operant conditioning, while started by Thorndike, was really refined by B. F. Skinner, who is considered the father of behaviorism. Again, we talked about behaviorism's fall during the cognitive revolution, but you can still see how much Skinner's operant conditioning permeates society today, including in the smoking cessation arena (and Quitters, Inc.!).

Let's discuss the basics of operant conditioning. While classical conditioning is all about learning automatic behaviors, operant conditioning is about learning behaviors through rewards and punishments. In a way, classical conditioning is something that occurs unconsciously; operant conditioning is more intentional. In operant conditioning, what happens after a behavior is performed is very important. When someone does something, the reaction of those around them will determine if they do that thing again or not. We have two main categories of what can occur after a behavior: (1) the behavior can be reinforced – that is, something occurs that will make the person more likely to do that behavior in the future, and (2) a punishment, which will make it less likely that the person will do that behavior in the future.

Both reinforcement and punishments have different flavors. For reinforcement, you have positive reinforcement – where you add something pleasant into the mix after someone does something – so giving a reward. You can also have negative reinforcement – that is you take something unpleasant away in response to a behavior. Here is a pigeon example: if you want a pigeon to do something, like peck at a certain color button, you can give them food as a reward for when they do it (positive reinforcement), or you can have loud, unpleasant noises playing, and when the pigeon pecks that button, the sound goes away (negative reinforcement).

Punishment also has a positive and negative component. Positive punishment involves adding something unpleasant to decrease a behavior, and negative punishment involves removing something pleasant to make the behavior less likely to occur. Back to pigeons – when you want to make sure the pigeon does not peck at the button, you will give them a shock every time they do (positive punishment) or you remove the food from their cage when they peck it (negative punishment). It is through using these forms of reinforcement and punishment, under multiple conditions, that you can train a pigeon to do almost anything – from delivering lifesaving messages during wartime, to dropping bombs![2]

You may start to see where this is going in terms of smoking cessation and *Quitters, Inc.* Contingency contracts and contingency management are both methods that leverage operant conditioning to help people quit smoking. Contingency contracts are formal documents written up by the person trying to quit and their therapist (sound familiar?), and it outlines specific goals and the rewards and/or punishments for not meeting those goals. Contracts can be part of contingency management but are not required.

In both contingency contracting and management, it is common for there to be a reward (vouchers or prizes) when a participant doesn't smoke (positive reinforcement) (Secades-Villa et al., 2020). Often, they do not go by patient self-report of whether they smoked or not, but they will use objective measures, like a breath test that detects carbon monoxide levels indicative of smoking. If the participant has a negative carbon monoxide breath test, they will then get vouchers for different items or experiences, or a cash equivalent. Studies will also look at cotinine levels, which we discussed in Chapter 6.

For the most part, operant conditioning-based contingency interventions focus on the reinforcement aspect. By providing incentives when a person hasn't smoked (positive reinforcement) or making it clear what negative aspects of their life are improving (not smoking is being rewarded by the removal of that hacking cough, or the bad smelling breath, a form of negative reinforcement), these programs are much more successful, especially in the short-term initial phases of quitting (Secades-Villa et al., 2020).

What doesn't seem to work so well is the punishment side of things. It seems that for a lot of people, especially if they are addicted to a substance, the negative consequences do not lead to change. Brand and colleagues (2025) state that this may be due to punishment insensitivity. Substance users may have already become used to the negative consequences of their habit, so any additional negative consequences may not faze them. It may also be that with their reward systems so altered by the substance, the rewards seem to outweigh the punishments.

⚠ **[Spoiler Alert]** However, this isn't quite the case with Jimmy and Dick. The horrifying negative consequences for others mostly win out over the rewards of smoking. For Dick, there is only one time that the potential rewards of smoking that cigarette get the better of him, and that is when he is stuck in terrible traffic. This is not surprising. One study by Shiffman (2005) used ecological momentary assessment (EMA) to see what was happening to people during the moments that they relapsed after quitting smoking. EMA is a research method where you collect data at several assessment points throughout the day, so that you can get a better moment by moment sense of what is happening. In this study, they found that smoking relapses were more likely to occur when the person experienced substantial increases in negative affect right before. An incident that could cause increases in feelings of frustration, anger, irritability, misery, sadness, and tension is likely to lead to smoking relapses. A traffic jam in the Midtown tunnel could definitely fit that bill!

Fortunately for Dick (and his wife and child!), the contingency contract he wrote with Vic Donatti does the trick – and his smoking days are far behind him (we hope).

Cognitive Behavioral Therapy – Not So Fast Behaviorism!

What if the extreme contingency contract that Dick entered into didn't work? What then? Chances are, if he had survived, he would have moved on to motivational interviewing (MI) and Cognitive Behavioral Therapy (see Chapter 9 for history of CBT).

Based on our review of the models of behavior change, it seems that both Jimmy and Dick had the behavioral intention (motivation) to quit smoking. But if they were on the fence, we might have to employ some techniques to get them over their ambivalence. MI is one of those techniques, and it involves active and empathic listening, helping people see what goals in life could be better achieved if the behavior change was made, and providing them with a sense of self-efficacy around their ability to achieve desired changes. It is very much NOT the way that Quitters, Inc. goes about the initial stages of their therapeutic intervention!

Once the person is ready to begin the work of change, CBT may be the next step. Since we are talking about how thoughts (the cognitive) and our actions (the behavioral) interact, this involves a lot of challenging the negative thought/behavior cycle. The participant and therapist may try to figure out what the triggers of the smoking behavior are and restructuring negative thoughts that enhance those triggers (e.g., "I can't get through an entire workday without a cigarette"). Work may be done on figuring out some relaxation techniques to cope with those triggering thoughts or events, or finding things to substitute for smoking, like exercise. There are many other components of CBT that may be used. CBT itself is very prescribed, but components can be modified for individual needs. CBT has been shown to be moderately effective, its effectiveness is enhanced when combined with other methods, such as contingency management (McHugh et al., 2010).

Conclusion

In the end, though, both Jimmy and Dick were successful with the Quitters, Inc. plan. Yet quitting could potentially be a lifetime struggle. One study that followed a group of smokers for approximately three years found that it may take more than 30 quit attempts for it to stick (Chaiton et al., 2016). Of course, those study participants weren't working under a contingency contract with Vic Donnati – and lucky for them, since no one has that many fingers and toes to spare!

Night Shift

Short Story Collection: King, S. (2011). *Night Shift*. Random House.
Audiobook: King, S. (2016). *Night Shift* (W. Patton, Narr.) [Audiobook]. Audible Studios. https://www.audible.com
Movie: Teague, L. (Director). (1985). *Cat's Eye* [Film]. Dino De Laurentiis Company; Embassy Pictures.

Further Explorations

1 We only touched upon a few of the more widely known theories of behavior change in this chapter. One we did not get a chance to discuss was the transtheoretical model of behavior change (Prochaska & Velicer, 1997). This model

was developed specifically to address addictive behavior like smoking, and it involves stages of change. The stages are:

1 Precontemplation – here, the person has no desire to change their behavior, and they may not even know that their behavior is problematic. People in this stage have little or no incentive to change.
2 Contemplation – here is where people start being aware that they have a problem and may start thinking about changing a behavior to solve it. However, they are only thinking about it – they have not yet taken any steps to start working on the behavior.
3 Preparation – this is when the person has set an intention to change. They may be changing small aspects of their behavior, but they have not yet made the full commitment.
4 Action – at this stage, the person is actually changing their behavior. They are putting their energy and activity toward making a significant change in the behaviour.
5 Maintenance – this is when the behavior change has been made, and actions must now shift to keeping the change in place and preventing relapses (which can send a person back to any of the previous stages).

After reading *Quitters, Inc.* – can you describe either Jimmy McCann or Dick Morrison's journey through the transtheoretical stages?

2 In 1985, Lewis Teague directed a movie called *Cat's Eye* that was an anthology of three Stephen King's short stories. *Quitters, Inc.* was the first story presented, and Dick Morrison is played by James Woods. There are two parts in the movie that vary slightly from the text, and they are worth looking at from a health psychology perspective. First is the appearance of the waiting room of Quitters, Inc., and what appears on the walls – anti-smoking posters. The second is a party that Dick Morrison attends, where EVERYONE is smoking (even the kids!).

First, the posters in the waiting room are using fear appeals – the assumption being that if you make people afraid, they will make the changes to reduce the fear. Search the literature – do fear appeals work? What else might be needed to make it effective? What public health campaigns have been successful in educating you about the dangers of smoking?

Next, watch the party scene. What psychosocial factors can you see at play? Will these make him more or less likely to relapse?

Notes

1 See Chapter 6 for more about secondhand smoke, also called environmental tobacco smoke (ETS).
2 Yes, Skinner led Project Pigeon – his attempt to train pigeons to drop bombs during WWII (the US military discontinued the project in 1944). Luckily, pigeons are much better at delivering messages, which have actually saved countless lives. Pigeons have even won military awards for their service – like Cher Ami, the pigeon who won the French Croix de Guerre after being injured while delivering a message to American troops in WWI. He was also posthumously awarded the Animals in War and Peace Medal for Bravery.

Bibliography

Ajzen, I. (1991). The theory of planned behavior. *Organizational Behavior and Human Decision Processes, 50*(2), 179–211

American Lung Association. (2023). *Overall smoking trends*. Retrieved October 26, 2025, from https://www.lung.org/research/trends-in-lung-disease/tobacco-trends-brief/overall-smoking-trends

Brand, M., Müller, A., Wegmann, E., Antons, S., Brandtner, A., Müller, S. M., … & Potenza, M. N. (2025). Current interpretations of the I-PACE model of behavioral addictions. *Journal of Behavioral Addictions*, *14*(1), 1–17. https://doi.org/10.1556/2006.2025.00020

Chaiton, M., Diemert, L., Cohen, J. E., Bondy, S. J., Selby, P., Philipneri, A., & Schwartz, R. (2016). Estimating the number of quit attempts it takes to quit smoking successfully in a longitudinal cohort of smokers. *BMJ Open*, *6*(6), e011045.

Christakis, N. A., & Fowler, J. H. (2008). The collective dynamics of smoking in a large social network. *New England Journal of Medicine, 358*(21), 2249–2258.

Davidson, K. W., & Scholz, U. (2020). Understanding and predicting health behaviour change: A contemporary view through the lenses of meta-reviews. *Health Psychology Review*, *14*(1), 1–5. https://doi.org/10.1080/17437199.2020.1719368

Dyal, S. R., & Valente, T. W. (2015). A systematic review of loneliness and smoking: Small effects, big implications. *Substance Use & Misuse*, *50*(13), 1697–1716. https://doi.org/10.3109/10826084.2015.1027933.

Eelen, P. (2018). Classical conditioning: Classical yet modern. *Psychologica Belgica*, *58*(1), 196. https://doi.org/10.5334/pb.451

Hajek, P., & Stead, L. F. (2001). Aversive smoking for smoking cessation. *Cochrane Database of Systematic Reviews*, (3). https://doi.org/10.1002/14651858.CD000546.pub2

Jolma, C. D., Samson, R. A., Klewer, S. E., Donnerstein, R. L., & Goldberg, S. J. (2002). Acute cardiac effects of nicotine in healthy young adults. *Echocardiography, 19*(6), 443–448.

Kassel, J. D., Stroud, L. R., & Paronis, C. A. (2003). Smoking, stress, and negative affect: Correlation, causation, and context across stages of smoking. *Psychological Bulletin, 129*(2), 270–304. https://doi.org/10.1037/0033-2909.129.2.270

Kim, K., & Picciotto, M. R. (2023). Nicotine addiction: More than just dopamine. *Current Opinion in Neurobiology, 83*, 102797. https://doi.org/10.1016/j.conb.2023.102797

King, S. (2012). *Night Shift*. Random House. https://www.amazon.com/dp/B0078XGJXO

King, S. (2020). *On Writing: A Memoir of the Craft* (25th anniversary ed.). Scribner. https://www.amazon.com/dp/B08CVP2HXP

Le Foll, B., Piper, M. E., Fowler, C. D., Tonstad, S., Bierut, L., Lu, L., … & Hall, W. D. (2022). Tobacco and nicotine use. *Nature Reviews Disease Primers*, *8*(1), 19.

McHugh, R. K., Hearon, B. A., & Otto, M. W. (2010). Cognitive-behavioral therapy for substance use disorders. *The Psychiatric Clinics of North America*, *33*(3), 511–525. https://doi.org/10.1016/j.psc.2010.04.012.

Prochaska, J. O., & Velicer, W. F. (1997). The transtheoretical model of health behavior change. *American Journal of Health Promotion, 12*(1), 38–48. https://doi.org/10.4278/0890-1171-12.1.38

Razali, M. F. (2025). History and evolution of E-cigarettes. In Y. H. Leong & A. S. Mohd Samin (Eds.), *E-Cigarettes* (pp. 1–12). Springer. https://doi.org/10.1007/978-981-96-5087-3_1

Rosenstock, I. M. (1974). Historical origins of the health belief model. *Health Education Monographs*, *2*(4), 328–335.

Saha, S. P., Bhalla, D. K., Whayne, T. F., & Gairola, C. G. (2007). Cigarette smoke and adverse health effects: An overview of research trends and future needs. *International Journal of Angiology*, *16*(03), 77–83.

Secades-Villa, R., Aonso-Diego, G., Garcia-Perez, A., & Gonzalez-Roz, A. (2020). Effectiveness of contingency management for smoking cessation in substance users: A systematic review and meta-analysis. *Journal of Consulting and Clinical Psychology*, *88*(10), 951–964. https://doi.org/10.1037/ccp0000611

Shiffman, S. (2005). Dynamic influences on smoking relapse process. *Journal of Personality*, *73*(6), 1715–1748. https://doi.org/10.1111/j.0022-3506.2005.00364.xDigital Object Identifier (DOI)

Society for Health Psychology. (2023). *About*. https://societyforhealthpsychology.org/about/

Tweed, J. O., Hsia, S. H., Lutfy, K., & Friedman, T. C. (2012). The endocrine effects of nicotine and cigarette smoke. *Trends in Endocrinology & Metabolism*, *23*(7), 334–342. https://doi.org/10.1016/j.tem.2012.03.006

U.S. Department of Health and Human Services. (2014). *The health consequences of smoking—50 years of progress: A report of the Surgeon General*. U.S. Department of Health and Human Services, Centers for Disease Control and Prevention, National Center for Chronic Disease Prevention and Health Promotion, Office on Smoking and Health. https://www.hhs.gov/sites/default/files/consequences-smoking-exec-summary.pdf

Wold, L. E., Tarran, R., Crotty Alexander, L. E., Hamburg, N. M., Kheradmand, F., St. Helen, G., … & American Heart Association Council on Basic Cardiovascular Sciences; Council on Arteriosclerosis, Thrombosis and Vascular Biology; Council on Hypertension; and Stroke Council. (2022). Cardiopulmonary consequences of vaping in adolescents: A scientific statement from the American Heart Association. *Circulation Research*, *131*(3), e70–e82. https://doi.org/10.1161/RES.0000000000000544

11 Done Is Done

Where We Are and Where We Go

But that's enough. Fun is fun and done is done.

(King, 2002, p.470)

Thank you for following me on this journey. It is a very interesting juxtaposition when we are talking about the evidence-based science of health psychology with the mysterious and unknowable world of Stephen King. I would like to state here that while I am a scientist by training, and the scientific method is at the core of what I teach, I still like to leave room open for the unexplainable, for the magical, for the beyond knowing. I think that this is an important facet of being human. I hope that this book has left you open to both the knowable and the unknowable.

A Message to the Audience

In the preface to this book, I mentioned that it was written for three main audiences: those who want to learn about health psychology, those who want to teach health psychology, and Constant Readers. I would like to address each of you as we come to the end of this book.

Those Who Want to Learn about Health Psychology

We have certainly covered a wide range of health psychology topics, and I hope that you have enjoyed learning about new things or reviewing what you already know. Yet we haven't even begun to scratch the surface of all that health psychology is. Some important topics still to explore:

- Chronic disease management and psychological adjustment
- Adherence to medication
- Nutrition
- Exercise
- Social support
- Loneliness
- Cultural Impacts

DOI: 10.4324/9781003495994-11

- Environmental and climate factors
- Health literacy
- Mindfulness
- Pain and pain management
- And on and on and on,

The point is not to say what a lousy job I did covering all that health psychology entails, or to make you feel like you didn't really learn anything about health psychology. The point is to say – keep going! There are so many exciting things out there to learn about and study further – the health psychology field is your oyster!

If you found something that really piqued your interest, or something that you can see yourself wanting to get further involved in, there are many avenues for pursuing your health education further. There are also many careers within the field of health psychology; you may find one that is right for you. Let's go through just a small sampling of your options, based on what interested you the most in this book.

Public Health

Did you find that you were really excited when we talked about the epidemiologist's bathtub? What about infectious disease surveillance? Or coming up with interventions addressing smoking cessation? If yes, then a career in public health might be for you. You could become an:

- Epidemiologist – study the patterns and etiology of diseases.
- Biostatistician – work on the statistics dealing with relative risks, twin concordance rates, and other health data.
- Health Educator – design programs that make use of the Health Belief Model, or Theory of Planned Behavior to promote healthy lifestyles.
- Environmental Health Specialist – interested in the kind of environmental factors discussed in *The Running Man*? This position would allow you to study environmental risks that impact population health.
- Public Health Policy Analyst – have a role in creating those larger system policies that we talked about with Bronfenbrenner's ecological model.
- Disaster Response Coordinator – be ready when Captain Trips lands.
- And so much more!

If you are an undergraduate student, and any of this sounds up your alley, I would highly suggest looking into an MPH (master's in public health) program. Getting my MPH was one of the best decisions I have made in my life. It provides you with real-world, marketable skills that can easily get you on the path to a very successful career in public health.

Health Psychology Research

If you found you were more engrossed in our discussions of the research methods, the way that studies are designed and conducted, and how we can use the results to interpret our world, you may want to focus more on research careers, such as:

- Research Assistant/Research Coordinator – handles recruitment, data collection, and all the other essentials that make research run.
- Lab Technician – work on experimental setup and equipment.
- Data Analyst – analyze the data using statistical software such as R and SPSS.
- Program Evaluator – use research skills to develop assessments for programming across the psychology and health spectrum.
- And so much more!

From personal experience, you can definitely get many of these positions right out of undergraduate study. Finding an MPH program that is focused on research can also further train you in program assessment and statistics. There are also plenty of master's programs that focus solely on biostatistics. If you are interested in doing your own research one day, then you will want to start thinking about Health Psychology PhD programs.

Clinical Health Psychology

Maybe what excited you most was the idea of providing cognitive behavioral therapy to someone suffering from insomnia or trying to quit smoking. Maybe you would like to assess psychopathology or help those experiencing suicidality. In that case, it sounds like you are more interested in the applied, clinical side of health psychology. There are lots of options out there:

- Behavioral technician – implement interventions and collect data on particular patient populations.
- Health program coordinator – work on developing and delivering community health programs.
- Hospital Social Worker/Oncology Social Worker/Transplant Social Worker/Emergency Department Social Worker – the list goes on and on in terms of the types of social workers who serve in the medical and health realm.
- Clinical Health Psychologist – focus on behavioral interventions, helping clients with chronic illnesses, and so forth.
- And so much more!

For behavioral technicians and, in some cases, health program coordinators, all that is needed is an undergraduate degree. An MSW (master's in social work) is required for the wide range of medical and health-related social work positions. Clinical psychology will require a PhD.

No matter what you are interested in, you can do this! The world needs more health psychology, and you can see evidence of that every day. So do what you can to learn as much as you can, and I will see you out there in the field. Maybe we could even discuss some Stephen King when we see each other!

Those Who Want to Teach Health Psychology

I hope that this book has inspired you – reminded you how much you love the topic of health psychology, and how much fun it is to come up with new ways to address it within your classroom. After each chapter, I have provided questions that you can use as assignments or discussion topics within your class. Within each chapter, I have also provided information about audiobooks, TV shows, miniseries, and movies that can be substituted in for the books, should you find assigning reading something like *The Stand* too much of a burden for your students.

Of course, you do not have to assign the entirety of all the novels discussed here. Let's take *The Stand*, for example – you could just assign the first third of the book, which is really the most health psychology relevant. The same with *It* – you could assign those relevant Eddie Kaspbrak chapters.*Quitters, Inc.* and *The Body* are relatively short reads to begin with. My sense, though, is that if you are going to assign your students many pages of reading, they would probably prefer it to be Stephen King, then say *The Way of an Investigation* by Walter Cannon. But I could be wrong!

I have also designed this book so that it easily aligns with many of the introductory health psychology textbooks out there. I have also provided you with some generic rubrics, which can be found on the eResource section of this book's product page on www.routledge.com/9781032802077. Please feel free to use and shape them however you would like. They are designed to go with most of the "Further Exploration" questions at the end of each chapter – either via a written assignment or a class discussion.

I also sincerely hope that this helped you find your own inspiration for creating out-of-the-box assignments. Maybe there is a favorite author you would like to introduce to your students and use to illustrate the topics you are most passionate about. I say go for it! Maybe it is not an author, but a TV show, or a TikTok series, a graphic novel, or manga (I am thinking about *Moyashimon*, which has characters based on microorganisms; Ishikawa, 2009). There are so many things that we can do to keep ourselves and our students excited about the material – Stephen King was able to do it for me – what about you?

Constant Readers

Did you enjoy learning all about health psychology while getting your Stephen King fix? I certainly hope so, as that was one of the goals I had in the back of my mind while writing it. I love when I can multi-task – learning both about Stephen King and the biopsychosocial model is really a win-win for everyone! You may also have noticed that there were a lot of things I left out for the sake of brevity (something that King himself is not very good at). There is also still so much of King's world left to explore. For example:

- *Duma Key* – the biopsychosocial factors involved in recovering from a brain injury (King, 2008).
- *The Dark Tower* series – exploring heroin addiction through Eddie Dean, looking at the impact of race on health and disability through Odetta Holmes (King, 1982–2012).
- "The Man Who Would Not Shake Hands" – further investigating placebo and nocebo effects through this short story from *Skeleton Crew* (King, 1985).
- *Rose Madder* – understanding the physical and psychological correlates of domestic violence (King, 1995).
- *Bag of Bones* – the impact of complicated grief (King, 1998).
- And on and on and on

You have probably made your own connections to other works while reading this – please reach out and share (or meet me on the Stephen King reddit page, r/stephenking). We still have so much to talk about! But for now, I wish you all long days and pleasant nights.

References

Ishikawa, M. (2009). *Moyasimon: Tales of agriculture* (Vol. 1). Del Rey Manga.

King, S. (1982–2012). *The Dark Tower series*. Various publishers.

King, S. (1985). *Skeleton Crew*. Putnam.

King, S. (1995). *Rose Madder*. Viking.

King, S. (1998). *Bag of Bones*. Scribner.

King, S. (2002). *Dreamcatcher* (Kindle ed.). Scribner. https://www.amazon.com/dp/B000FBFN1U

King, S. (2008). *Duma Key*. Scribner.

Index

Note: **Bold** page numbers refer to tables; *italic* page numbers refer to figures and page numbers followed by 'n' refer to notes.

For Product Safety Concerns and Information please contact our EU representative GPSR@taylorandfrancis.com
Taylor & Francis Verlag GmbH, Kaufingerstraße 24, 80331 München, Germany

www.ingramcontent.com/pod-product-compliance
Ingram Content Group UK Ltd.
Pitfield, Milton Keynes, MK11 3LW, UK
UKHW020006200926
475702UK00015B/2507
9781032802077